THE THEOLOGENIC DIET

WHAT THE BIBLE SAYS ABOUT DIET, HEALTH, & NUTRITION

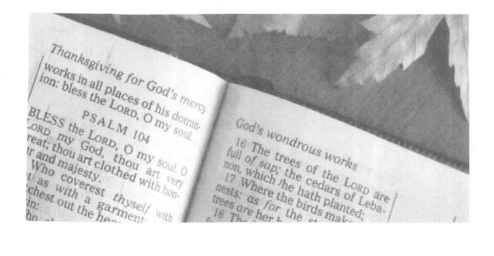

By Rebecca M. Austin

The Theologenic Diet
By: Rebecca Austin (Coach Green)
Healthy Homestead Living
A division of Strive 4 Savvy, International S.A.
©2018 Strive 4 Savvy International S.A.
First Edition

Cover design done by Denise Barringer, Maddix Publishing
Title page design done by Strive 4 Savvy, International
Typesetting, book layout, compilation, photography, and publishing done by Strive 4 Savvy, International. All photographs used in the book are either the property of Strive 4 Savvy, International, used with permission, or public domain.

All Bible quotes have been taken from the YouVersion Bible App. More information about this free app can be found at YouVersion.com or in your app store.

Published by: Strive 4 Savvy, International & Maddix Publishing
Edited by: Strive 4 Savvy, International, & Maddix Publishing

ISBN: 978-1-7326471-0-7

Disclaimer: As with any diet changes, additions, or substitutions it is recommended to use good judgment and if need be ask for the advice of your healthcare provider. The author of this book is not a certified nutritionist, nor healthcare professional. The ideas, concepts, and opinions expressed in this book are intended to be used for educational purposes only. None of the information provided is intended to offer medical advice of any kind, nor is this this book intended to replace medical advice, nor to diagnose, prescribe, or treat any disease, condition, illness, or injury.

Author and publisher claim no responsibility to any person or entity for any liability, loss, or damage caused or alleged to be caused directly or indirectly as a result of the use, application, or interpretation of the material in this book.

Acknowledgements:

First, I'd like to thank my Father God who is always with me. He put it on my heart to write this important message and guided me throughout the process. God's people are getting sicker and sicker, but it is when we are well that we can best live the lives we are meant to live.

Nothing could have happened in this book or any of my projects without all the love, patience, and sacrifices of my husband, Andy. Thank you for all your support and working so hard so I could focus on writing.

Special thanks go out to my guiding light and driving force, my beautiful and talented daughter Megan. You give me so much purpose. Your smile, your hugs, and your laughter never cease to bring me such peace and joy.

I wouldn't be where I am today without the wisdom and love of my dear mom, Joyce. I miss you every day and look forward to the day I get to see you again in Glory.

Sincerest gratitude goes to my friend and mentor, Dawn Roller, who always has such a big heart for people and who always knows when to push me a little harder to strive a little higher. Success never comes without incredible support through a powerful Inner Circle and I am so blessed you saw something in me that at one time I didn't even see in myself. We've come a long way since those first days at the university, yet even then God had bigger plans for both of us.

A word of thanks to my mentors, Tamara Lowe with Kingdom Builders Academy, and James Wedmore with Business by Design. Your encouragement and your willingness to push me a little harder to stretch outside my comfort zone have helped me grow in ways I never knew were possible. Through your guidance I have come to embrace the discomforts, overcome the fears, and learn from the failures, so I can do what God intends for the benefit of others. You are all truly anointed and I am so blessed to work under your tutelage.

To all my followers on my website **www.healthyhomesteadliving.com,** my blog, my social media pages and my videos, I offer my biggest thanks. For without you, Healthy Homestead Living would be nothing more than an idea. Thank you for all your comments, feedback, shares, discussions, and love that keeps me going; always looking for bigger and better to share with you so you can live a life of peace, joy, harmony, and abundance.

God Bless.

Rebecca Austin (Coach Green)

Contents: Biblical Steps to Health

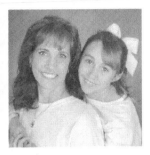

INTRODUCTION:

A year ago, I never thought I would spend the next several months writing this book, and I don't consider myself a well-versed theologian. I do love learning about food and eating healthy, have studied healthy living concepts for most of my life, and I consider myself a devout Christian. I am a homesteader, a master gardener, a wife, a mother, and a lover of good, nourishing foods. When God put it on my heart to write this book, however, I did what most of us do when God tells us to do something; I questioned His choice. "Why me Lord?"

I grew up on a farm in rural Wisconsin. We had a large garden every year, raised a few cows, goats, sheep, chickens and horses, with much of what we ate coming from our own labor. As a small child, I just took it for granted that everyone understood where our food comes from, how it grows, how to preserve it for the winter months, and how to cook without prepackaged convenience. As I got older I started to become more aware of the changes in our culture and how food was becoming less about health, nutrition, and survival and more about convenience, economics, social satisfaction, and self-gratification. We have developed into a culture that centers around food; but not necessarily for nourishment.

From the time we are toddlers we are "rewarded" with food, bribed with food, distracted with food, and educated with food. Birthdays, holidays, and celebrations center around the table. Social outings revolve around dinner out and a movie with more food. Business meetings are often held over coffee or lunch. We are conditioned to turn to food when we are depressed; seeking out our "comfort foods". Our emotional and

AND GOD SAID:

1 Corinthians 10:31

So whether you eat or drink, or whatever you do, do all to the glory of God. (ESV)

Philippians 3:19

Their end is destruction, their god is their belly, and they glory in their shame, with minds set on earthly things. (ESV)

psychological approach to food has drastically drifted as a culture from what God originally intended. Too often we fall into habits that God warned us about in Philippians 3:19 with, "Their end is destruction, their god is their belly, and they glory in their shame, with minds set on earthly things." (ESV) or in Psalm 78:18, "They tested God in their heart by demanding the food they craved." (ESV) We put our cravings over God, self-indulging to the detriment of our health and our relationship with God.

On top of that, our physical approach to food has drastically changed over the years to focus on mass production, big business, complex marketing strategies, and attention to profits. Companies started genetically modifying what used to be healthy ingredients. Family farms started disappearing, being replaced by vast farms that deplete the soil, encourage erosion of the precious topsoil, and require more and more chemicals to maximize yields.

As a result, overall, we are getting sicker and sicker. Obesity is a serious problem. Cancer, heart disease, strokes, and diabetes continue to rise as top health concerns. And most heartbreaking of all is the rise in childhood issues that were rare when I was a kid; health problems like childhood diabetes, attention disorders, autism, food allergies, and worst of all, childhood cancers.

Despite all this, when God first nudged me to write this book, I didn't feel at all qualified and immediately started giving excuses why I shouldn't write this book... "I don't know enough about Your Word, Lord"... "Who am I do give this message?"... "I am not eloquent enough"... "Who would want to listen to me anyway?"...

But God kept nudging me and I found verses floating off the pages of the Scriptures when I was in the Word... or at church... or even scrolling through social media; verses about life, health, and abundance... verses about food and what God intended us to eat to thrive. We are, as a whole, getting sicker each passing decade and the need to turn back to God's guidance for our health and well-being is becoming more and more crucial. God wants us to be WELL! God wants us to THRIVE!

When we are well, we can do so much more in His kingdom. Wellness of body, mind, and spirit. When we are well, we have more peace, more energy, more drive and can impact others so much more positively. We can help others, encourage others, and uplift others so much more. Conversely, when we aren't well, we lack the energy or the motivation to do much of anything. Our bodies and our minds are more focused on trying to get better or on just surviving than on impacting the world or making a difference. Something compelled you to pick up this book and start reading it. Deep down in your spirit, you know that there are things you could change to improve your health. I encourage you to focus on health as your goal. The contents of this book are not designed as a weight-loss program, rather a lifestyle-of-health-through-God program. The great side-benefit of health, however, is your body will then naturally and more healthfully achieve its optimum weight.

God loves us so unconditionally and **He wants us to be well**. But He also loves us so much, that He gives us **free choice.** We can make our own decisions about every aspect of our lives, decisions which do have consequences. Through ignorance or intent, how we feed our body, our mind, and our spirit **will** affect our overall health and well-being. I encourage you to take a moment and prayerfully consider your current relationship with food. God says in 1 Corinthians 6 that our body is our temple in which the Holy Spirit dwells. In this book, I will share what it means for our bodies to be temples and what we can do to live a life of health, peace, prosperity, and abundance in Him; what it means to develop habits so you can thrive.

This book is the culmination of years of study and prayer with the intention to give you some insights so you can make choices that will impact your health in a positive way. The information provided may open your eyes and give you new insight into how God teaches us through His Word to be healthy. Yet, information won't benefit you without action and some amount of discipline to create new habits. These new habits can greatly impact your life in ways you may not even begin to imagine. You just need to get started and then create new patterns of health. And the great part is that we will guide you each step of they way, and our Heavenly Father will support you when you stumble, encourage you when you weaken, and rejoice with you when you succeed.

Most of what you read about biblical diets come from direct study of certain verses, then translating them to how that verse or verses apply to our daily lives. I took a much different approach in writing this book. The information offered here comes from scientific studies, personal experiences, both with my healing and my husband's battle and victory with cancer, and many years of study to learn the "why" behind healthy foods. I then took that information and applied it

AND GOD SAID:

Exodus 23: 25

Whorship the Lord your God, and his blessing will be on your food and water. I will take away sickness from among you, ...and I will give you a full lifespan. (AMP)

7

AND GOD SAID:

Hosea 4:6

My people are destroyed for lack of knowledge.

to what God says about health, diet, and nutrition. Most chapters have two sections: a section about our physical health and a section about our spiritual health. Health is a delicate balance between the physical, emotional, mental, spiritual, and physiological parts of our selves.

When looking at the Bible as a guidebook to healing and living healthy, it is important to look at all angles and find where we can improve; where we can draw closer to Him through His Word. Often the Bible is very literal and the message is clear; yet other times the interpretation is subjective and more philosophical, speaking to each individual on his or her terms. As you read through the chapters of this book, consider prayerfully how the information applies to you and your situation, **then seek professional guidance if needed.** None of the information provided is intended to replace the advice of your professional healthcare provider.

It is also important to consider that when it comes to our health, it is just as important what we feed our spiritual bodies as what we feed our physical bodies. Both must be fed regularly or we will wither and die. Sometimes, when we think we feel physical hunger, it is actually our spiritual bodies that are craving attention. For example, how often do we find ourselves turning to food during times of depression or stress? Therefore, to help you with both your physical and spiritual growth, I include in each chapter some spiritual guidance in reference to that topic, in additional to physical guidance according to God's Word. Please don't overlook this crucial point. Your health is a result of more than diet. It is the culmination of what you have fed yourself physically, yes... but also spiritually, emotionally, and mentally. For **true** health you must find balance in **all** areas.

I have no doubt that God has guided me carefully through each and every chapter in this book, and it is my prayer that you find value in the information provided.

The health industry is big business. You can't turn on any media without being bombarded with marketing slogans and colorful ads trying to get you to buy the latest, greatest supplement, exercise program, diet program, pharmaceutical drug, or "snake oil" that is going to fix your problems. Why are there always so many fad diets out there claiming to be the next greatest thing in our quest for weight loss and health? Fad diets that come and go...because they only work short-term, or don't work at all. I'm not saying that all programs or products are bad; just that we are consuming them from the wrong approach, and for the wrong reasons. If we look first to God for guidance in all things, then follow His plan with the right frame of mind and the right intentions, then He will bless us, support us, and guide us as to what is best for us. God has our best interests in mind. Big businesses do not.

It is my belief that everything I need to know about life is found in the pages of my Bible... including what we should be eating and how we should be living for optimum health. This book describes what I am calling the **"Theologenic Diet"**. God put this title on my heart one night, at about 2:00 a.m. when I should have been sleeping, but instead awoke with this clear message that He wanted me to share. "Theologenic" comes from the Greek root words, meaning "of God's logic".

This diet is not mine, rather God's guidelines. I do my best to share with you God's Logic, through God's Word, then the scientific "why" behind how those verses affect our bodies, our health, our immune systems, and our well-being.

As with any time spent in the Word, we all hear different messages at different times of our lives, depending on what we need to hear or learn at that time. I encourage you to seek out these verses. Do your own research about what I share. And spend some time communing with God, seeking His guidance for you and your health, both spiritually and physically.

The book is divided into three sections: The Healthy Body, The Healthy Lifestyle, and The Healthy Mind. For some of you, the guidelines offered here are a major change from your current lifestyle and may seem overwhelming. Let me encourage you to prayerfully consider each section and do your best to make a few changes at a time. Rome wasn't built in a day, and you can't expect your habits to change overnight. Take a few ideas that resonate with you and put them into action... then add more as time goes on. Follow the Action Items listed at the end of each chapter. Before you know it, you'll start seeing improvements... and it gets easier and easier to make adjustments for the better. Any action, in the right direction, is better than doing nothing... or worse, staying at the status quo. The key is to develop good habits according to God's direction using discipline and perseverance. God is with you and will help you through the times when you stumble. Keep trying. I believe in you.

May you find value in this book, health, peace, and joy that comes from our gracious Heavenly Father, through Christ Jesus. Amen.

Blessings,
Rebecca Austin (Coach Green)
HealthyHomesteadLiving.com
TheologenicDiet.com

AND GOD SAID:

Psalm 107: 20

He sent forth His word and healed them...

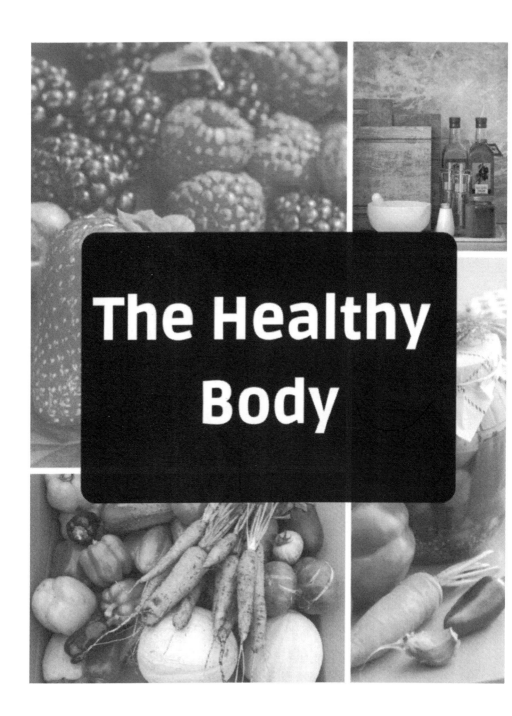

The Healthy Body

Chapter 1: Let There Be Light

The Physical Significance of "Light"

In the beginning, God said, "Let there be light."

Life begins with light. Light is energy and all living beings require energy to survive. Scientists have discovered that even the tiniest organisms and even bacteria use (and are made up of) energy. So, we can confidently say that the foundation for all life is energy. On earth, the source of our light and energy comes from the sun. Spiritually, our light and energy comes from the Son.

Health is all about energy and light, which is why we begin with light in the first chapter of this book, just as God started the universe with light. Whether it be spiritual health, physical health, or mental health we can heal through energy and through light. As we journey through these pages together, I will often refer back to energy and light and how they relate to our health.

The term "light" can refer to several aspects of our health. First, there is the physical light that comes from the sun. This is the energy that is transferred to us either from direct absorption such as the vitamin D we get from being in sunshine, or it could be the energy we get from consuming foods that contain energy stored from sunshine.

For example, plants use a process called photosynthesis to convert energy from the sun. During photosynthesis, the energy from the sun is combined with water molecules that have been absorbed through the roots and then converted into food for the plants. Excess energy is stored as chlorophyll which is the substance that gives leaves their green color.

Animals who eat plants convert the chlorophyll into energy, and excess energy is stored as fat. The closer you get to the original energy from the sun, the more nutrient-dense that energy source becomes. This is why most "diets" recommend plant-based nutrients over animal-based nutrients, particularly your leafy greens. Eating more greens is one of the few diet recommendations that almost all "diets" will agree upon. We'll discuss this in more detail later in our chapter on vegetables, fruits, leafy greens, and microgreens.

AND GOD SAID:

Genesis 1: 3-4

And God said, Let there be light; and there was light.
And God saw the light, that it was good: and God
divided the light from the darkness. (ASV)

Luke 11: 34- 36

Your eye is the lamp of your body. When your eyes are healthy, your whole body also is full of light and healthy. But when they are unhealthy, your body also is full of darkness. Therefore, if your whole body is full of light, and no part of it dark, it will be just as full of light as when a lamp shines its light on you. (NIV)

Essentially, every core function in our bodies, from cell regeneration to movement, brain function, digestion, emotional responses, and everything in between require energy which either comes directly from the sun or indirectly from the sun through the foods we eat.

Obviously, this is a very basic overview of an incredibly complex system involving scientific studies such as biology, biochemistry, bioengineering, botany, ecology, genetics, evolutionary biology, hematology, and many others, yet it gives you the overview of the importance of light energy in our physical health. When we understand how important light is in creation and in God's plans for us, we can approach many foods with a different understanding, particularly when choosing which foods are most important to consume regularly for optimum health.

In modern diets, the norm has become the consumption of primarily "convenience" foods, which unfortunately, consist of mostly dead foods; foods that have all the energy and life processed out or cooked out. These foods are manufactured for ease of preparation, economics, and mass distribution. Very little thought has been put into preserving any of the life-force or energy in these foods. Coupled with the number of added sugars, unhealthy salts, and chemicals added to give those foods back some semblance of flavor, we have a highly toxic substance. Worse, since our bodies are not given the nutrients it craves for the energy it needs, we are still hungry. Thus begins a vicious cycle:

- We eat dead foods...

- Dead foods contain sugars, unhealthy salts, and chemicals that make us crave them more...

- Sugars, unhealthy salts, and chemicals make our bodies work harder, causes inflammation, feeds bad bacteria and harmful organisms in our bodies, and depletes our inner resources...

- Our bodies are still hungry due to still not getting the nutrients and energy it needs to thrive so craves more...

- We eat more dead foods.

The good news is that this cycle can easily be broken by simply adding living foods back into the equation. This means consuming whole foods that still have as much life-force from the sun's light energy as possible. We'll share greater insights on the specifics of these foods and how best to prepare them according to God's plan in the subsequent chapters, but before we do it is important that you understand the beauty of God's design for abundant life, a life that comes from light and energy. A few examples of powerful living foods with the most light energy include:

- Leafy Greens like Kale, Lettuce, Beet Greens, Swiss Chard, Collards, etc.

- Microgreens and Sprouts

- Vegetables and Fruits (Raw, Lacto-fermented, or lightly cooked)

- Nuts, Seeds, Legumes, and Whole Grains (soaked)

- Herbs

- Sea Vegetables

- Mushrooms

- Cultured Dairy

- Kombucha, Kvass, and other probiotic-rich beverages

- Cultured (Lacto-Fermented) Foods

Science has proven that living foods such as those listed above are higher in vitamins, minerals, micro nutrients, amino acids, enzymes, phytonutrients, probiotics, and prebiotics than most other foods on the planet. These are also the foods that most efficiently store the life energy or light from the sun. In some circles, these foods are referred to as "superfoods".

Feed your body with light and feel the difference. When I first started eating more living foods, I found myself craving them. I grew up on a farm so was very familiar with fruits and vegetables so these foods weren't anything new... but regularly consuming "superfoods" like sea vegetables, microgreens, sprouts, and cultured foods was new to me. I was surprised how much I enjoyed them. The more I ate

AND GOD SAID:

James 1:17

Every good and perfect gift is from above, coming down from the Father of the heavenly lights, who does not change like shifting shadows. (NIV)

AND GOD SAID:

Ephesians 5:8

For at one time you were darkness, but now you are light in the Lord. Walk as children of light. (AMP)

them, the more I loved the flavors and the more I appreciated how much better I felt! You may even surprise yourself, too.

The Importance of Sunshine to Health

God gave us the light from the Sun to benefit us more than just by what we can consume through living foods. Our bodies need sunshine just as much as plants do. Sunshine on the skin converts a form of cholesterol just under the skin into vitamin D, an important vitamin crucial to the body's ability to assimilate and metabolize calcium into the body. Sunshine also helps the body balance pH, kill fungus and bacteria, and is one of the ways the body regulates serotonin, the mood hormone.

As our traditional lifestyles convert to outdoor labor and children playing regularly outside to one of sedentary hobbies, indoor jobs and activities, and an increase of electronics, an alarmingly rapid increase of vitamin D deficiency is being seen in young and old alike. This deficiency gives root to other serious health conditions including brittle bones, immune disorders, and neurological disorders. Getting outside, enjoying some sunshine, and supporting the body in a way God designed it will significantly support healthy vitamin and mineral absorption.

Too much sun is not good for the body in that it can cause burns, acidic conditions, and dehydration; however, too little sun will eventually deplete the body of crucial balances. Specialists recommend a minimum of 15 minutes a day of sun exposure, particularly to the face, for optimum vitamin D exposure and absorption. In the case of fair skin or easily burned skin, start with shorter times and slowly work your way up to longer periods as your skin adjusts. Babies need sun too, so don't be afraid to let them enjoy some rays, always being careful to avoid over exposure.

As for sunscreens, most commercially available lotions are loaded with harmful chemicals that are more toxic and harmful to the body than over exposure to the sun would be. When in the sun for longer periods of time, use wide-brimmed hats, protect the skin with long, loose clothing, and/or choose a natural lotion that doesn't have all the toxins.

Light as a Therapy for Physical Healing

Light from the sun is made up of different spectrums of wavelengths, each producing what our eyes see as different colors. NASA researchers found in the 1970's that a certain wavelength of near infrared light penetrates about 2.5 centimeters into the body's tissues, with a myriad of benefits. For over 20 years, scientists have been conducting clinical research on photonic red light therapy with astonishing results. Researchers in published medical studies have found that photonic red light therapy:

- Reduces pain by increasing endorphin production, a natural pain killer.

- Reduces inflammation by suppressing enzymes that create swelling, redness, and pain, and boosts the release of anti-inflammatory enzymes.

- Stimulates the mitochondria within the cell, increasing ATP production. Increase of ATP allows damaged cells to accept nutrients faster and to better eliminate toxins.

- Increases lymphatic drainage

- Increases circulation to the area and triggers communication with the brain for faster healing

- Increases antibody production in the blood stream to allow the body to fight off viruses.

- Relaxes tight muscles and quickly releases muscle cramps.

- Increases collagen production, a protein vital to tendons, bones, skin, teeth, and cartilage.

- Regulates serotonin levels. Serotonin plays an important role in blood clotting, stimulating a strong heart beat, initiating sleep, and fighting depression.

Photonic red light therapy has been effective in both humans and animals to support healing with an estimated 50% faster healing times. God created so many wonderful tools at our disposal to support health and healing! (*A) Other light

AND GOD SAID:

John 8:12

When Jesus spoke again to the people, he said, "I am the light of the world. Whoever follows me will never walk in darkness, but will have the light of life." (NIV)

Matthew 5: 13-16

You are the light of the world. A city that is set on a hill cannot be hid. Neither do men light a candle, and put it under a bushel, but on a candlestick; and it gives light unto all that are in the house. In the same way, let your light shine before others, that they may see your good deeds and glorify your Father in heaven. (NIV)

wavelengths, such as certain blue, green, and ultraviolet lights also have been found to have healing qualities. For more information about how photonic red or other colors of light therapy might benefit you, visit www.PhotonicLightTherapy.com.

The Spiritual Significance of "Light"

Spiritually, "Light" plays a significant role in God's Word. First, light represents a "brightness" in our souls and in our spirits.

The word "Light" is associated with images of brightness, happiness, love, peace, joy, togetherness, and all things good. Even as small children we are taught to "let our light shine." One of my favorite Sunday School songs is "This Little Light of Mine, I'm Gonna Let it Shine." (You'll have that song in your head now for a couple days.... You're welcome. :-) It is such a happy song and uplifts my spirit. I hope it does yours, too.)

"Light" is the opposite of "dark," yet it is also the opposite of "heavy". When we carry the light of the Lord inside of us, our inner light glows brightly for all around us to see through our joy, patience, understanding, helpfulness, thoughtfulness, and generosity. The brighter our inner light, the closer we draw to Him and the more we represent the Glory of God to others. This inner "light" comes from the presence of the Holy Spirit that resides within us.

I was at a a church event several months ago. The venue was packed and there were over 10,000 people attending. My friends and I had trouble finding a seat. When we finally got settled, several of my friends were grumbling about how frustrated they were and how annoying it was to deal with such a crowd..., when suddenly I heard the most joyful giggle coming from the lady next to me. I turned to her and she gave me the most radiant smile you could possibly imagine. I smiled back and she leaned over and whispered in my ear, "What a blessing to be at such an amazing place with so many people worshipping our Heavenly Father!" Her joy in just being there was so evident and so beautiful. She had the option to get grumpy about the crowds, the difficulty in finding a seat, the venue, or any number of other "complaints," yet instead chose to let her inner light shine. And that radiant light warmed all those around her, including me.

What a difference it would make in our world if more would understand this simple concept and allow the light of the Lord to shine through them. That's not to say that we don't have times when we hurt, are "heavy" with the world's problems and pains, but I have learned that when I find my inner light starting to dim, all I have to do is turn to Him and He adds oil to my lamp so my light can shine brighter once again. And often, this brightness starts with a prayer and a smile.

Here's a fun little exercise for you. Take a moment and smile. Allow your smile to brighten your whole face. Really get into it. How does that make the rest of you feel? Lighter? Happier? More energetic? Smiling is a wonderful way to lift your spirits when you feel low and will often help you feel lighter, happier, and even more energetic. Laughter is even better!

Guess what? When you smile with an inner light at another person, that energy is transferred to the other person. Too often in the hustle and bustle of this modern, technological world we live in where people are communicating more through phones or computers, we miss out on so many opportunities to truly connect with others. A smile is a wonderful gift you can give another... and the side benefit is it adds to your own light energy when you do! Unfortunately, smiling through an emoji just isn't the same.

Try it for yourself and experience the wonder of sharing God's inner light that is inside of you with the world.

Another spiritual approach to "light" is that Jesus is the source of Light Himself. In John 8:12, Jesus says "I am the light of the world. Whoever follows me will not walk in darkness, but will have the light of life." Just as we physically get our light energy from the sun, we cannot underestimate the importance of how we spiritually get our light energy from the Son.

All that is good, all that is positive comes from the Lord. In 1 John: 5-9 we learn:

> "This message we have heard from him and declare to you: God is light; in Him there is no darkness at all. If we claim to have fellowship with him and yet walk in the darkness, we lie and do not live out the truth. But if we walk in the light, as He is in the light, we have fellowship with one another, and the blood of Jesus, his Son, purifies us from all sin."

Turn to Jesus to feed your spirit with the light your soul needs for deep nourishment. He is the source of our spiritual life-giving energy and light.

AND GOD SAID:

Psalm 27: 1

The Lord is my light and my salvation; whom shall I fear? The Lord is the defense of my life; whom shall I dread?

Chapter Summary

Life begins with "Light". The physical self and the spiritual self relies on light as the foundation of energy and vitality. Physical energy and vitality comes from the sun, primarily through consuming living foods that nourish. Spiritual energy and vitality comes from the Son, primarily through fostering a relationship with Him on a daily basis. To become truly healthy, we must consider and respect the importance of light/energy in our lives.

Action Steps:

Knowledge is power and the first step to seeing positive results comes from awareness and knowledge. However, knowledge is worthless without action. I heard it said by an amazing mentor, Caleb Maddix, that the key to results is Information + Application = Transformation. You must add action to the mix to see any improvements in your life. Each chapter, we will give you some suggested actions steps to take to start developing healthier habits and see the best results.

Action steps to start doing NOW:
1. Become aware of how much "light energy" you are consuming in your foods. What are you currently eating that is "dead" and what are you eating that is giving you "life"? What is on your plate that is nourishing and has sun energy? Keep a log for at least a week to increase your personal awareness of your current eating habits.
2. Start adding more foods with "light energy". Increase your intake of leafy greens, vegetables, sprouts, nuts, and fruits and try avoiding foods that are overly processed and "dead".
3. Spend some time outside in the sunshine, starting slowly if needed to allow your skin and body to adjust. Tilt your face up to the sun (avoiding direct sunlight in the eyes) and give thanks to God for the healing light He provides.
4. SMILE. Increase your inner light through regularly monitoring your attitude and how much your inner light is allowed to shine through to others.
5. Share a smile with others and find humor in situations as much as possible. Spread the light energy to those around you.

Notes:

Use this space, and the space offered after each chapter to map out your action items, thoughts, prayers, or whatever else God puts on your heart. The physical act of writing something down helps your mind absorb the information better. I love jotting down thoughts in the pages of the books I read as it helps me organize my thoughts; and I find it insightful to read those notes at later dates. My Bible is quite colorful with favorite verses highlighted and notes in the margins. My cookbooks have lots of notes about recipe alterations and family reactions. Feel free to turn this book into an interactive guide. This is your page!

Chapter 2: Breath of Life

Physical Significance of "Breath"

Our independent lives begin with our breath. Before that, we are a part of our mother, safe in the womb, relying on her for our nourishment, care, and support. Once we are born and draw our first independent breath, we are now our own person. The breath is the foundation for life itself. Scientists say that the average person can survive about 3 weeks without food, 3 days without water, and 3 minutes without breathing. The breath is the cornerstone to life itself and without it, our body systems quickly start to shut down, starting with the brain.

When God created Man, life began with God's Breath. In Genesis 2:7, we read about how God created man and then breathed into his nostrils the breath of life. Our very existence began with breath. But what exactly happens when we breathe, and why is our breath so important to life and to health?

The Breath, particularly oxygen, is crucial to every cell in the body. Molecular oxygen (O_2) is responsible for converting food into energy, cell regeneration, building of new tissue, replacement of old tissue, metabolism, reproduction, and just about all activities that we characterize as "life."

The average adult, by mass, consists of 65-90% water (H_2O, which is hydrogen and oxygen) and close to 100 trillion cells, each designed to perform an essential life function. Ninety-nine percent (99%) of the mass of the human body is made up of only six primary elements: oxygen, carbon, hydrogen, nitrogen, calcium, and phosphorus with oxygen composing the majority at 65% of the body by mass. All other elements are important yet in significantly smaller quantities such as potassium, sulfur, chlorine, sodium, magnesium, iron, zinc, iodine, selenium, cobalt, and fluorine, to name a few. (*2)

With a complete lack of this crucial element of oxygen, our brains would cease to function, our cells would collapse, and we would quickly die. However, what is happening to many of us in our modern world of indoor activities with stale air, sedentary lifestyles of sitting for long periods that constrict our diaphragm and reduce deep breathing, increase of pollution and toxic environments, and increased stress which causes the body to naturally take shallow breaths, is that we may be getting enough oxygen to survive but not enough oxygen to thrive. When we do

AND GOD SAID:

Genesis 2: 7

Then the Lord God formed a man from the dust of the ground and breathed into his nostrils the breath of life, and the man became a living being. (NIV)

not receive enough oxygen, we may become fatigued, lethargic, depressed, restless, prone to chronic illness, develop circulation issues such as cold hands and feet, experience dizziness, have headaches, see an increase in blood pressure, and a wide array of other symptoms and issues. (*3)

Many of us are suffocating slowly and don't even realize it. Because we need oxygen on a cellular level and for life itself, how we breathe, the quality of the air we breathe, and the amount of breath that gets into our system will affect our over-all health on a very deep level. Just reading this, do you have the urge to yawn? Drawing your brain's focus and attention to your breath and your breathing often results in the desire to yawn or take a couple deeper breaths.

Breathing is not something we normally have to think about. Our brains take care of controlling this action on auto-pilot... but that doesn't mean that we are always getting enough oxygen for optimum health. Sometimes we have to consciously take back over and breathe with intent.

As a kid, a fun game my siblings and I would often play was the yawning game where we would randomly try to get people around us to yawn. We would be at a family gathering, at church, at friends' houses or anywhere with a group of people and yawn... then see how many people we could get to yawn, too. Then we would giggle with each other over how many people we got to yawn, keeping score of who got the most reactions. Just reading this, did you find yourself yawning or experiencing the urge to yawn?

Here are a few ways you can ensure you are getting enough deep breathing each day to give your body the oxygen it needs:

- Start the day when you first wake up with a few deep breaths and a deep stretch.

- Add yoga to your routine. Yoga is a practice of focusing on breath, becoming mindful, and stretching, which is a wonderful way to reduce stress, center the mind, and breathe.

- Open the windows when you can at your house, office, and car to allow fresh air to circulate or if you live in an area with high levels of pollution, use an air purifier or air filtration system so your environment has fresh rather than stagnant air.

- Avoid breathing polluted air whenever possible.

AND GOD SAID:

Job 32:8

But it is the spirit in a person, the breath of the Almighty, that gives them understanding. (NIV)

3 John 1:2

Beloved, I pray that all may go well with you and that you may be in good health, as it goes well with our soul. (ESV)

- Watch your posture when seated to allow for deeper breathing and if you have to be sitting for long periods of time, take regular breaks to stretch and breathe.

- If needed, check with your healthcare provider to test your oxygen levels and see if supplemental oxygen might be beneficial for you.

I remember when I first started learning and practicing meditation. Before that, I had the misconception that meditation was a pagan practice and that it had no bearing in my life. In reality, even Jesus meditated, and through meditation we are quieting the mind, focusing on our breath, and communing with God. My first time meditating, I was amazed at how peaceful and relaxed I was, and yet at the same time, how energized I felt. If you don't already meditate regularly, I recommend you give it a try.

Another aspect of breath and oxygen in our physical health comes from what happens when pollution, radiation (including wifi), cigarette smoke, herbicides and chemicals, among other disrupters cause what we call "free radicals."

To understand free radicals, we have to once again go back to science and how the body is comprised. Our body is made up of cells, which are composed of different types of molecules. Molecules consist of one or more atoms of elements, like oxygen, joined by chemical bonds. Atoms consist of a nucleus, neutrons, protons, and electrons. When atoms bind together, they sometimes gain, lose, or share electrons. Sometimes, these bonds leave an unpaired electron which then leads to a free radical.

Normally, the body can handle free radicals, and in some cases such as when fighting a virus, free radicals are beneficial. If free radicals present in the body become excessive, however, damage can start to occur.

To reduce the effects of free radicals in the body and for optimal health, it is recommended to reduce your exposure to external causes as mentioned earlier, if at all possible, and to be sure to consume living foods that are rich in antioxidants. "Antioxidants" are defined as "molecules stable enough to donate an electron to a rampaging free radical and neutralize it, thus reducing its capacity to damage." (*5) Foods high in antioxidants include:

- Vitamin C foods such as citrus, kiwi, strawberries, bell peppers, and broccoli.

- Vitamin E foods such as almonds, avocados, and olives.

- Beta-carotene and Vitamin A foods such as carrots, sweet potatoes, kale, chard, and papayas.

- Lycopene foods such as tomatoes, papaya, and watermelon.

- Lutein and zeaxanthin foods such as dark green leafy veggies such as spinach, kale, collard greens, and broccoli.

- Anthocyanin foods such as blueberries, raspberries, plums, pomegranates, eggplant, and red cabbage.

- Other antioxidant foods such as onion, garlic, cinnamon, curry, turmeric, cumin, holy basil, fenugreek, and ginger. (*6)

We will talk more about these foods in later chapters, but it is important to include them in this chapter when we talk about breath, oxygen, and health. Oxygen gives us life, yet when free radicals become too excessive, adding healing foods to our diet will allow our bodies to find balance and to heal.

The Spiritual Significance of "Breath"

The word "Spirit" comes from a translation of a Hebrew (and Greek) word that means "breath" and at other times "wind." Often in scripture, when we read about the Breath of God, we are talking about the presence of the Holy Spirit.

"Spirit, then, is something forceful or powerful. The Holy Spirit, the holy breath of God or wind from God, brings with him God's power. He enables what he enters into to operate with spiritual or divine power. That is why Jesus said in Acts 1:8, "But you shall receive power when the Holy Spirit has come upon you," and why Peter said in Acts 10:38, " God anointed Jesus with the Holy Spirit and with power." (*7)

It is through the Breath of God, the divine Holy Spirit which resides within each of us, that we are given the ability to connect with God on a much deeper level through greater wisdom and understanding, sound judgment, empathy, peace, and a deep abiding love and appreciation that only comes from our Heavenly Father.

AND GOD SAID:

1 Corinthians 3: 16-17

Do you not know that you are God's temple and that God's Spirit dwells in you? If anyone destroys God's temple, God will destroy him. For God's temple is holy and you are that temple. (ESV)

23

Job 12: 10

In his hand is the life of every creature and the breath of every human being. (NIV)

Our physical bodies must be fed regularly so that we have strength, endurance, energy, and life. In order to be healthy, we must make good choices in how we care for our physical bodies such as diet, exercise, rest, and avoiding stress. Our physical body is referred to in the Bible as our temple; a temple in which the Spirit resides. For optimum health, we must not only feed our physical bodies with good food; we must also consider what we are doing to feed our spiritual bodies.

Our spiritual bodies must be fed just as much, if not more so, than our physical bodies. Without feeding our spiritual bodies every day through prayer, mediation, communion with God, fellowship, worship, music, and praise, our spiritual bodies become weak; making us susceptible to darkness, negativity, depression, longing, doubt, hopelessness, and so many other dark forces and emotions.

I can speak from experience on how important it is to feed your spiritual body and to stay connected with the Holy Spirit within. Shortly after I graduated from college I found myself drifting from my Christian roots. I was young and out on my own for the first time in my life. I had my own apartment, found a decent job that helped pay the bills, and had very few responsibilities. Life was fun... at least for awhile. But I quickly started to feel restless. I thought I was doing pretty well, at least compared to others my age. I had no college debt, I drove a car that was paid for, I had a savings account, and I wasn't going hungry. But I was too "busy" to go to church due to my work schedule. I stopped volunteering because I had too much other stuff to do. I wasn't spending time with God regularly; essentially I was living a me-centered life. I thought I was happy, but I was lonely, often confused, completely lacked self-confidence, and relied too heavily on what others thought about me for my sense of self-worth. Major decisions were made by calling my "friends" and asking their opinions first, rather than asking God.

When I finally came to my senses and turned back to God, I was overwhelmed by the intensity of how full my spirit felt; exemplifying the emptiness that was there before. I was washed in such powerful peace, grace, love, and humility and my eyes were once again opened; yet clearer than ever before, on God's amazing love and grace. It is only through feeding our spiritual bodies by drawing closer to God the Father, God the Son, and God the Holy Spirit that we can truly find optimum health. It is through the Holy Spirit that we find strength, joy, peace, compassion, hope, fulfillment, and love.

Chapter Summary

We all need to breathe to survive because oxygen is required for so many important life functions. Even when breathing, however, we may not be getting enough oxygen to thrive. Our lifestyles, pollution, physical challenges, inactivity, and other factors may be contributing to our slow suffocation, affecting our overall health.

Spiritually, the Breath of God resides within us in the form of the Holy Spirit. It is just as important for us to focus on our spiritual selves as it is to look at our physical selves when seeking health and abundance. True health can only come from a balance of both the spiritual body and the physical body.

Action Steps:

What actions will you start taking to improve your Physical and your Spiritual Breath of Life? Here are a few suggestions to help you get started.

Actions items to start doing NOW:

1. When you first wake up in the morning, take several deep, cleansing breaths. Breathe by expanding your diaphragm downward rather than raising up your lungs or shoulders. Feel the breath fill your whole body. Repeat throughout the day as necessary, especially when you feel tired.

2. If you find yourself sitting for long periods of time, watch your posture so you still have the ability to breathe deeply and take regular breaks to stretch and breathe.

3. Practice yoga regularly.

4. Avoid chemical exposure, pollution, and toxic air whenever possible. Don't leave your cell phone on the bedside nightstand when you are sleeping so you aren't exposed to the harmful WiFi and radio waves while your body is resting and healing.

5. Make it a priority to feed your spiritual body (prayer, worship, meditation, praise music, etc.)

6. Avoid feeding your spirit with too much negativity such as violent or graphic movies, negative media, negative people, angry music, etc.

Notes:

Chapter 3: Life-Giving Water

No guidance about health would be complete without taking time to emphasize the importance of drinking water and getting sufficient hydration; and the Bible, as our ultimate guide, references water 722 times!

In the Bible, water represents many things. At times, water in scripture represents health and hydration. Other times, water is mentioned when discussing cleansing or cleanliness (more on that in Chapter 13). Some verses refer to water as the very word of God, and others use water to even represent life itself.

The first mention of water can be found in Genesis 1:2, the last in Revelation 22:17, with water flowing throughout the pages of scripture in between these two books like a river, winding us through scripture on a journey of God's Word. (*8)

Let's take a quick look at each of these representations, how they affect us today, both physically and spiritually, and what we need to know for optimum health.

The Physical Significance of Water

Water has always fascinated me, at least since my middle school years when I first learned in science class about the periodic table and how atoms of these key elements interact. Scientifically, water is made up of two gases that are bound together by an electron: two hydrogen atoms and one oxygen atom (H_2O).

Water is one of the only substances on the planet that can exist in all three physical states; liquid, solid, and gas depending on temperature. If the Earth, whose surface is roughly 70% water, were any closer to the sun, then life could not survive as the water would primarily be a gas. Similarly, if the Earth were any further from the sun then life could not survive as the water would primarily be ice. It's no coincidence that God placed us exactly where He did in the Universe, the perfect distance from the sun for the perfect balance of temperatures for water to exist in primarily liquid form and sustain life.

Physically, our bodies are made up of approximately 65% water, with higher concentrations in the brain (73%), heart (72%), lungs (83%), and kidneys (79%). Water plays a significant role in our bodies by helping regulate body

AND GOD SAID:

Exodus 23: 25

You shall serve the Lord your God, and He will bless your bread and your water. And I will take sickness away from the midst of you. (AMP)

Revelation 22: 1

Then the angel showed me the river of the water of life, bright as crystal, flowing from the throne of God and of the Lamb. (ESV)

temperature, protecting the spinal cord and brain, lubricating and cushioning joints, aiding in digestion and elimination of waste, and hydrating the cells. Our blood, tissues, organs, and bones all need water to function and thrive. Basically, every major function in your body needs hydration through water.

Water has the unique ability to dissolve other substances; so much so, that a steady dripping of single drops of water can dissolve rock, creating deep canyons and vast caves. Have you ever witnessed the sheer magnitude of the Grand Canyon or toured the beautiful caverns of the Mammoth Cave? This fascinating ability of water to dissolve is also the key to dissolving nutrients internally so they can be distributed to the cells in our bodies for nourishment.

And, that's not all. Water also has the ability to distribute and absorb heat without drastically affecting its core temperature. Without this amazing quality, we wouldn't be able to survive in the extremes of nature that humans live. Since our bodies contain primarily water, our inner body temperature remains relatively stable. A fluctuation of as little as 8° could be fatal. Similarly, because our bodies are primarily water, our bodies can self-regulate higher core temperatures as needed in the form of a "fever" to fight off viruses and bacterial infections that threaten the well-being of the host. This heat distribution ability also makes water the best remedy for burns.

God created water, with all these wonders that seemingly defy the science of other elements, to support life to its fullest. We need pure water for optimum health. In fact, there are a surprising number of "ailments" and "diseases" that can be remedied quite quickly just by giving the body sufficient hydration. An estimated 80% of the U.S. population is dehydrated to some extent and drinking enough water can alleviate, and in some cases even reverse, constipation, digestive disorders, skin disorders, high blood pressure, brain fog, insomnia, chronic fatigue, and depression.

Our bodies are constantly using and eliminating water through the lungs, kidneys, skin, and colon with an estimated daily loss averaging around 2 liters, or about ½ gallon. Consumption of caffeinated beverages, soft drinks, and alcohol further dehydrates the body. Specialists agree that for the body to stay fully hydrated, we need to consume half our body weight in ounces each day at a minimum, under normal activity levels. This amount would increase with physical labor or activities done out in the sun. For example, an adult weighing 180 pounds should consume at least 90 ounces of water each day (around ¾ gallon).

Quantity of water is one thing to consider, yet quality of water is also important. Please note that when we discuss drinking water to stay hydrated, this is in the form of pure water. Other beverages like herbal tea, kombucha, kvass, kefir, and other healthy drinks are great and should by all means be consumed regularly; however it's best to add these beverages above and beyond your daily water requirements. Beverages such as soft drinks, alcohol, processed drinks, or chemically flavored drinks should be avoided as they stress the body and in many cases, actually contribute to dehydrating the body. Drink pure water for best results. When Jesus walked among us, water was pretty simple. The Bible references water as purest in the form of dew or from springs, and also references the rivers, streams, brooks, and oceans. Modern times of commercialism, pollution, and technology have created a confusing array of choices for where we get our water. Let's take a quick look at a few of these choices and which are best.

The Best Water Choices For Regular Consumption:

Well Water
Well water is generally considered a good source of healthy water, since well water comes from drilling down to a natural water source deep below ground and often contains beneficial minerals. However, well water typically does not go through regular testing for harmful bacterial levels or hard minerals like iron. If you live in an area that utilizes well water, have the water checked for safety and adjust accordingly using in-home filtration systems or water purification systems as needed.

Natural Spring Water
Spring water is pure, clean water that flows from a natural spring and is bottled at the source. If you buy natural spring water, be aware that some companies claim to be selling natural spring water but regulations allow a "mixture" of natural spring water and other water so it may not be pure. Also be aware if it's bottled in plastic that certain plastics can leech into the water, essentially contaminating the contents.

Artisan Water
Artisan water is natural spring water that is bottled somewhere other than the source and is generally processed and purified. Same cautions apply. Watch for the plastics and buy from a reputable company.

AND GOD SAID:

Deuteronomy 33: 28

Jacob's spring is secure in a land of grain and new wine, where the heavens drop dew. (AMP)

29

Proverbs 5: 15

Drink water from your own cistern, flowing water from your own well. (ESV)

Ionized Water

Ionized water is water that has been filtered and then electrolyzed to create water that has either more alkaline or more acidic pH. There is no conclusive evidence that electrolyzed water has specific health benefits, but there are many people who swear by it. Ionized water, however, has no documented negative effects either, so it makes our "good" list.

Acceptable Water Choices:
Use Sparingly, Occasionally, or with Caution

Reverse Osmosis

Reverse Osmosis water has been run through fine membranes that purify the water by removing large particles, pollutants, and minerals. Made popular by larger companies such as Culligan, offering drinking water convenience to offices and homes, reverse osmosis water is one of the best-tasting water choices available. The downside, and the reason reverse osmosis made our "use sparingly" list, is because the process of reverse osmosis is so effective that you are left with literally nothing but pure H2O. As a result, scientific study is now showing that prolonged effects of drinking reverse osmosis water can create mineral deficiencies in the body. Mineral deficiency can lead to things like migraines, high blood pressure, insulin resistance, constipation, and even heartbeat irregularities. Drinking reverse osmosis can be moved to the "good" list if you add a mineral supplement to your regimen.

Distilled Water

Distilled water comes from vaporizing the water, leaving behind heavier substances like pollutants and minerals. Like reverse osmosis water, the result may not have pollutants, but because it also doesn't have minerals, it can lead over time to mineral deficiencies. Again, if you decide to drink distilled water, be sure to supplement with the necessary minerals to keep your body healthy.

The Worst Water Choices: Avoid Whenever Possible

Tap Water

Tap water refers to the water that comes from the faucets of most modern homes. If you live in the city, tap water has been processed, purified, stored, and transported to your home. Processing, to comply with EPA guidelines, often involves adding chlorine to kill bacteria and aluminum sulfate to coagulate organic particles. The water is then put into a settling bin to allow the coagulation to settle, then is filtered, treated with lime to adjust the pH, and in some areas infused with fluoride, before it is sent to storage reservoirs. (*9) Despite the Safe Drinking Water Act that was signed in 1974 to help regulate municipal water, most tap water is not recommended as a healthy option for regular consumption. The addition of chemicals and the levels of pollutants still found in most homes' water makes tap water an undesirable choice.

Bottled Water

Believe it or not, a large majority of the bottled water companies just purify tap water and then market it. What you are paying for is the bottling, transporting, and marketing. It takes an average of 1.63 liters of water to make every liter of Dasani, according to one study; and bottling companies are depleting the natural water resources from thousands of communities around the globe. (*10) The plastic from the bottles can leach into the water in them creating a beverage that is costly and unhealthy. Add to that the environmental effects of the plastic bottles in the trash after you are done with them, and we have the "least" of the options.

In summary, the best water you can drink is pure, clean, mineral rich water that comes from a natural source and is enjoyed in glass, stainless steel, or other sustainable, reusable, and recyclable material. Water is one of the most important elements of a healthy lifestyle, so make sure you are choosing the best whenever possible, and consuming enough to fully support the many functions in the body that need water to thrive, namely at least half your body weight in ounces.

When I first started tracking how much water I was drinking each day, I was surprised at how far off I was from getting enough water for my body. Without realizing it, I was drinking about half of what I should have been. Focusing on this one healthy habit, within a very short time I saw huge improvements in how I felt. My dry, cracked skin started healing, I was sleeping better, I felt less tired, and I had better focus. If you don't think you like the taste of water, try adding some fresh cucumber, fresh strawberries, other fresh berries, sliced lemon, and/or fresh herbs like basil, lavender, or mint; creating a delicious and refreshing beverage.

Another important physical aspect of water is cleansing. Personal hygiene is very important to our health. Often we read in the Bible, particularly in passages in

AND GOD SAID:

1 Samuel 30: 11-12

Then they found an Egyptian in the field, and brought him to David; and they gave him bread and he hate, and they let him drink water. And they gave him a piece of a cake of figs and two clusters of raisins. So when he had eaten, his strength came back to him; for he had eaten no bread nor drunk water for three days and three nights. (NKJV)

Yet whosoever drinketh of the water that I might issue him should never thirst; however the water that I should issue him might be in him a well of water springing up into everlasting life. (KJV)

the Old Testament about "clean" and "unclean". Some of these references were physical and others were spiritual yet both warrant further study and discussion. God's Word offers many verses with instruction on cleanliness. Sprinkled throughout Exodus, Leviticus, Numbers and Deuteronomy are various instructions concerning the washing of pots and utensils (Lev. 11: 32-35), clothes and bedding (Lev. 14: 8), a person's body (Lev. 15: 2-7, 22: 5-6), and recommendations regarding sanitation (Deut. 23: 12-14). (*11)   We know now, in our age of modern science, that many diseases and illnesses stem from viruses and bacteria that we can avoid with proper washing. Keeping our bodies, our homes, and our environments clean has a huge impact on pests, insects, parasites, and diseases. Bathing helps our bodies to eliminate toxins, improves our general sense of well-being, and helps us to be more pleasant to those around us. Isaiah 1: 16 instructs us to wash ourselves and make ourselves clean. We will dive deeper into cleansing in Chapter 13.

The Spiritual Significance of Water

Not only is water significant in our physical health, but Water is used many times in the Bible to represent important spiritual connections. At times, water represents spiritual purification, spiritual deliverance, spiritual cleansing, God's blessings, and at times even represents the very Word of God.

God uses water during significant times of spiritual deliverance in powerful ways. In Genesis 7, we learn how God cleansed the entire earth from evil by sending the great flood that covered the earth. In Exodus, we read the story of Moses and how first he was rescued from death as a baby by being hidden in a basket in the river; then how he led God's people out of Egypt by parting the Red Sea. Jonah was saved from death in the belly of a whale, despite his defiance to God's direction. Jesus' first "miracle" is found in John 2 when he transformed water into wine and Jesus defied the natural laws of earth by walking on water.

It is through baptism by water that we are washed of our sins and renewed in our spirit symbolically becoming dead to past sin, and then rising anew as pure through Christ and washed in the Holy Spirit.

Jesus himself is called the "living water". In John 4:14 we learn that it is through Jesus that our spiritual thirst is quenched forever. John 7: 38 says, "Whoever believes in me, as the Scripture has said, 'Out of his heart will flow rivers of living water.'"

With over 700 references in God's Word, both figuratively and literally, water plays a significant role in both our physical lives and our spiritual lives. It is through water that God's power and God's grace are revealed to us. Water reminds us of our creator, unites us with the Spirit, and purifies both the individual and the world.

Chapter Summary

Water is another foundational element, created by God, for life both physically and spiritually. Water is a cornerstone to our physical health through hydration of the cells, lubricating the brain, spine, and joints, dissolving and transporting nutrients, and so many other life functions. Water is also a cornerstone to our spiritual health. Jesus is called the "living water" and it is through Him that we find spiritual fulfillment, peace, contentment, and everlasting life.

Action Steps:

1. Drink half your body weight in ounces every day to maintain sufficient hydration and support your body. Increase this amount during times of strenuous exercise or when spending time outdoors where the body may be further depleted of hydration.
2. Practice good cleanliness and personal hygiene.
3. Turn to Jesus for spiritual cleansing. Spend time in the Word, in prayer, and prayerfully consider becoming baptized if you haven't already. Contact a pastor or church in your area if you have further questions in this area.

AND GOD SAID:

John 15: 3

You are already clean because of the word I have spoken to you.

Notes:

34

Chapter 4: Salt of the Earth

The Physical Significance of Salt

In recent years, salt has been getting a lot of bad publicity and many people believe that it is on the list of "unhealthy" foods that should be avoided. This is not the case, however. In reality, our bodies need salt to survive. Scientific research has not been able to show any evidence that eating a low-salt diet reduces the risk for heart attacks, stroke, or death. (*17) The **type** of salt **does** make a difference however, and consuming too little of the right kind of salt may be very detrimental; all of which we will discuss in great detail. Basically, it's important to distinguish between refined salt and unrefined salt; the latter of which is the preferred choice for health. Unrefined salt contains important trace minerals that complement the salt and accentuate the many benefits to the body. Become familiar with the differences between healthy salt and unhealthy salt, then make it a point to consume the right kind for your health.

Just as with water, salt is the combination of two elements: Sodium (Na), an unstable metal that can suddenly burst into flame, and chlorine (Cl), a lethal gas; joined together by an electron. When combined, these two elements form a substance that is essential for health and vitality. In the body, salt plays several major roles. First, salt, which is an electrolyte, acts as a link between intracellular fluid (the water inside your cells) and extracellular fluid (the water circulating outside the cells). This crucial link is how the body transports nutrients and hydration into the cell. This is why you can drink lots of water and still be dehydrated.

Salt also is a cornerstone to proper nerve function, contraction of muscles, including the most important muscle, the heart, and controls your taste, smell and tactile processes. (*13) It also aids in digestion, adrenal function, respiration and it helps the body maintain and regulate blood pressure. (*14)

Salt is generally found in nature in the ocean, large bodies of water fed by the ocean, or in areas that are now dried up but used to contain large bodies of water fed by the ocean. Let's take a quick look at the top types of salt, their impact on the body, and which is recommended for supporting health:

AND GOD SAID:

Job 6: 6

Can something tasteless be eaten without salt, or is there any taste in the white of an egg?

35

Leviticus 2:13

And every offering of your grain offering you shall season with salt; you shall not allow the salt of the covenant of your God to be lacking from your grain offering. With all your offerings you shall offer salt.

Refined Table Salt (Unhealthy... Avoid Whenever Possible)

Table salt, or refined salt, is the most common salt found on tables in America. If your doctor is telling you to reduce your salt intake, he/she is most likely referring to this type of salt. According to a recent study, Americans consume an average of about 10 grams of salt per day... but of this amount only about 20% comes from discretionary salt use, such as from the salt shaker. About 5% comes from sources such as water treatment and medications, and 75% comes from processed foods! (*15) The best way to cut unhealthy salts from your diet, therefore, is by cutting the unhealthy processed foods from your diet altogether, then making better choices for the remaining 20% to healthier salt options.

Refined table salt is made by collecting salt from mines or evaporated ocean water. It is then heated above 1200° F. Such a high temperature alters the chemical structure of the salt, making it difficult for the body to assimilate it as a needed substance. During this heating process, the other minerals present in the salt are stripped, and anti-caking agents in the form of dangerous chemicals such as ferrocyanide and aluminosilicate are added so that the salt will pour freely. This combination of heating, stripping of the natural minerals, and addition of toxic chemicals makes refined table salt a dangerous substance that harms our bodies.

Consuming too much table salt has been proven to cause high blood pressure, strokes, heart disease, stomach cancer, osteoporosis, kidney stones and kidney disease, vascular dementia, asthma, diabetes, mineral imbalances, and obesity... to name just a few. (*16)

Refined table salt has also been found to be a highly addictive substance. As with any drug, the body becomes accustomed to this fake sodium, and the more it has in the body, the more the body will crave it.

But, the good news is that all of the above listed harmful qualities are only the case with refined salts. Let's take a look at the healthier alternatives that God intended us to consume before we stepped in and tried to make God's creation "better" (aka, more economical for big business).

Celtic Sea Salt (Healthiest and Best Option)

Celtic Sea Salt is my personal favorite and preferred go-to salt for almost every culinary purpose. In addition, it is the only salt my doctor recommends to all his patients. Not only does Celtic Sea Salt taste amazing, but it contains lower ratios of sodium than other salts and contains the perfect balance of trace minerals including calcium and magnesium. Part of the reason my doctor recommends this salt, of all the other healthy salts listed in this book, it comes from an actual sea. Celtic Sea Salt originates from Brittany, France near the Celtic Sea so the salt itself is closest to a **true** sea salt. All other sea salts come from quarries that at one time were under water, often hundreds of thousands, and even millions, of years ago.

Celtic Sea Salt generally will be somewhat grayish in color and tends to retain more moisture so often will seem more "heavy."

According to medical studies, Celtic Sea Salt offers the greatest hydration to the cells, helps regulate blood pressure, supports digestion, encourages nutrient absorption into the cells, balances blood sugars, helps eliminate mucous buildup, builds the immunity, alkalizes the body, improves brain function, increases energy, and promotes a restful night sleep.

Himalayan Pink Salt (Another Healthy Option and Next Best)

Another great example of an unrefined healthy salt is Himalayan Pink Salt, also sometimes referred to as pink salt, Himalayan sea salt, and Himalayan crystal salt. Most commercial Himalayan Pink Salt comes from salt mines in Pakistan that are 5,000 feet deep below the Himalayan Mountain Range. Because these salt reserves have undergone tremendous pressure of millions of years, it is said this salt is over 99 percent pure, with variations of color from deep pink to almost red. The color variations in the salt come from the mineral content which is one of the qualities that makes Himalayan Salt a healthy salt choice for consumption. Not all Himalayan salt is the same, however, so be sure to choose only the best quality that comes from the deeper mines (more pure) rather than higher in the mountains (containing more pollutants).

Although personally, I prefer to use Celtic Sea Salt for my cooking and flavoring, I do love using Himalayan Pink Salt for several other uses in which salt is beneficial to health. Here are a few additional great ways to also use Himalayan Pink Salt other than direct consumption:

AND GOD SAID:

2 Kings 2: 21

And he went forth unto the spring of the waters, and cast the salt in there, and said, "Thus saith the Lord, I have healed these waters; there shall not be from thence any more death or barren [land]. (KJV)

Ezra 6: 9

Whatever is needed for a burnt offering to the God of heaven, and wheat, salt, wine, and anointing oil, as the priests in Jerusalem request, it is to be given to them daily without fail.

1. Salt Lamps. Salt lamps are from a large chunk of Himalayan Salt that has been semi-hollowed out to insert a low wattage light bulb. Salt lamps let off a charming glow, highlighting from the inside the beauty of the colors in the salt. The health benefits derived from the salt lamps are a result of the light which gently "heats" the salt. Salt in general is hygroscopic, which means it attracts water molecules. It is believed that Himalayan salt lamps contribute to purifying the air around it by attracting water molecules in the air that have indoor air pollutants like mold, bacteria, and allergens. Once in contact with the salt lamp, pollutants remain trapped and neutralized by the salt. Since the lamp is heated by the light inside it, the salt is allowed to dry, thus perpetuating this process.

Another benefit of salt lamps is their ability to reduce electromagnetic radiation in the form of unhealthy positive ions, which come from things like cell phones, computers, television, and other electronic devices. Himalayan salt lamps emit negative ions which cancel out the positive ions. Effects of electromagnetic radiation include fatigue, reduced immune system, increased risks of a variety of cancers, dementia, heart disease, and Alzheimer's disease. Using salt lamps to help neutralize the harmful positive ions are beneficial and many reports of better sleep, less stress, and fresher air have been reported. (*19)

Personally, I love my Himalayan salt lamps. I keep two large lamps in my bedroom and when the lights are on, you can definitely notice a difference in the freshness of the air in the room, much like when the window is open on a fresh spring day by the beach. If you decide to try them yourself, be sure to purchase a high quality lamp. There are many "knock-offs" in the market that won't offer the same results.

2. Bath Soak. It was Hippocrates, the father of medicine, who first discovered the healing qualities of salt, and throughout history, salt has been used medicinally and therapeutically. Soaking in a salt bath is not just for expensive spas. Some of the health benefits of taking a bath in Himalayan salt includes relaxation, detoxification, dermal mineral absorption, relief from aches, deeper sleep, therapy for skin ailments, respiratory relief, and increased circulation. For the salt bath to be the

most effective, you would want to add 1.28 ounces of salt per gallon of water in warm to hot water and soak for at least 20 minutes. (*18)

3. Pink Salt Scrubs. If you don't have time to soak in Himalayan Salt, try using it in a salt scrub. Salt scrubs detoxify the skin by penetrating deep into the pores of the skin pulling out dirt, pollution, and bacteria. The salt also exfoliates dead cells, balances skin pH, deodorizes, and tones the skin. You can easily make your own salt scrub by combining 1 cup of fine grain Himilayan Pink Salt with ½ cup of fractionated coconut oil, almond oil, or avocado oil. Add a few drops of essential oils if desired. Mix thoroughly and store in an airtight container. Use 1-2 tablespoons and scrub into the skin, being careful to avoid eye, nose, mouth, and ear areas.

4. Inhaler or Netti Pot. Since Himalayan Salt has been shown to improve symptoms of allergies, respiratory infection, asthma, sinus problems and coughs, adding Himalayan salt to a netti pot is a great way to support the immune system and respiratory system in a natural way. If you are unfamiliar with the Netti Pot, it is a small vessel in which you mix warm water and a saline or salt solution, then pour this mixture into one nasal cavity to drain out the other nasal cavity. This process flushes the nasal canal of toxins, pollutants, bacteria, and pathogens. If the thought of pouring salt water into your nose sounds too challenging, you can also use a salt inhaler, which basically is a small vessel filled with Himalayan salt and possessing a narrow opening with which the user gently places the lips around and breathes in deeply.

Some modern spas now have Himalayan Salt rooms, where the walls of the rooms are made of Himalayan Salt bricks. Sufferers of chronic respiratory issues greatly benefit from regularly breathing the salty air. Personally, I use Himalayan Salt Bricks in my Infrared Sauna for additional healing benefits while detoxifying. I'll share more on the benefits of using saunas in the chapter on detoxing.

5. Himalayan Salt Cooking Block. Salt cooking blocks are huge slabs of Himalayan salt used in food preparation or serving. Salt blocks add healthy minerals to the food, add a hint of salt flavor without too much, prevent the growth of bacteria and help "cure" the food through contact, and make beautiful serving platters that retain their temperature (either hot or cold) for a period of time.

AND GOD SAID:

2 Kings 2: 20

He said, "Bring me a new jar, and put salt in it." So they broght it to him.

AND GOD SAID:

Numbers 34: 12

And the border shall go down to the Jordan and its termination shall be at the Salt Sea. This shall be your land according to its borders all around.

As you can see, Himalayan Salt has many great benefits and uses, not only as a culinary ingredient but in medicinal remedies and personal hygiene practices. I encourage you to experiment for yourself to find what works best for you.

Redmond Real Sea Salt (Mineral rich, so also an acceptable choice)

Redmond Real Salt is also a sea salt that, like Himalayan Salt, comes from salt mines of ancient sea beds and is sold in its natural and unrefined state. As with Celtic Sea Salt and Himalayan Pink Salt, Real Sea Salt is mineral-rich and contains around 62 trace elements. Because Real Salt is mined in Utah in the United States, it can be readily found in many grocery stores in America and often has a much more economical price tag.

I use Real Salt while preserving vegetables from my garden. It works great for canning and for lacto-fermenting. The minerals in this salt give it a much milder flavor than Celtic Sea Salt or Himalayan Pink Salt. Because it only has 62 trace elements, where Celtic and Himalayan Pink have 82, Real Salt is not generally used in regular daily use in our home, however, as we tend to opt for the higher mineral options.

What About Other Salts?

There are many other salts on the market, too many for us to go into great detail in this book. The best rule of thumb in choosing a salt is to look at whether it is refined or unrefined and what the main purpose of the salt may be. For example, I'm often asked if kosher salt is considered a healthy salt. Kosher salt is a refined salt that has a much more coarse structure than table salt. Kosher salt got its name as a result of Jewish tradition in following God's law that meat be purified of blood before consuming (more on that in our chapter on meat) and coarse salts are more effective at extracting blood from meat while curing. Kosher salt is still refined, however, so not on our list of healthy salts. In fact, Celtic Sea Salt and Himalayan Pink Salt can be purchased in a coarser form making them preferred choices for curing meat.

Epsom salts are not actually salt but rather a naturally occurring mineral compound of magnesium and sulfate found near Surrey, England. Epsom salts are wonderful in medicinal remedies and in gardening, among other uses requiring magnesium in a bio- available form. I wouldn't use it to flavor my dinner, though.

Canning salt, or pickling salt, is a refined salt without any anti-caking additives or iodine. .
Some believe this salt is the best choice for preserving because without the anti-caking additives, the jars of green beans or pickles don't get cloudy as they would with refined table salt. Personally, however, I use an unrefined salt like Redmond's Real Salt and have never had a problem in all my years of canning.

When considering other salts not listed in this book, consider the source. Where did it come from? How was it processed? What is the mineral content? What will it do to my health? As long as you stick with salt that is unrefined and pure, you should have a salt that will benefit your health as God intended.

Iodine and Salt

Some theologians believe that salt and iodine are closely linked to the change in expected life span we see in the Bible prior to and following the Great Flood. Prior to the flood, it was not unheard of for man to live for several hundred years. After the fall and the Great Flood, where God cleansed the earth, the life span was reduced to 120 years. Prior to the flood, the earth was mineral-rich. Iodine levels in particular were considerably higher. After the flood, however, the levels of iodine were diluted; so much so that even today the best sources of iodine only come from the sea through seaweed, sea vegetables, and fish.

In 1924, iodine was added to refined table salt to address what was perceived as a deficiency of iodine in America. The amount of iodine found in modern refined table salt is so negligible, however, that it barely warrants labeling. Couple that with the dangerous side-effects of refined salt to the body, it is better to get iodine from more balanced sources including unrefined salts as mentioned or sea vegetables like kelp, nori, or dulse. Talk to a healthcare professional if you are curious about your iodine levels and whether you need supplementation.

Throughout history, salt has played a significant role in traditions, health, and wealth. Salt was used during biblical times as a currency, for seasoning food, for preserving food, for medicinal practices, and in rituals.

AND GOD SAID:

Numbers 18: 19

All the offerings of the holy gifts, which the sons of Israel offer the Lord, I have given to you and your sons and your daughters with you, as a perpetual allotment. It is an everlasting covenant of salt before the Lord to you and your descendants with you.

Ezekiel 16: 4

As for your birth, on the day you were born your naval cord was not cut, nor were you washed with water for cleansing; you were not rubbed with salt or even wrapped in cloths.

The Spiritual Significance of Salt

Symbolically, salt in the Bible represented hospitality, durability, fidelity, and purity. Mike Ford, in his essay about salt written in 2002, aptly entitled "Salt," describes the spiritual importance of salt the best. He wrote:

> *In antiquity, Homer called salt a divine substance. Plato described it as being especially dear to the gods. Today, we take salt for granted; we think of it as a common, inexpensive substance that seasons food and clears ice from roads.*
>
> *However, salt has many more amazing properties and uses. It seasons, cures, and preserves. It also seals, cleans, and acts as an antiseptic. In a booklet put out by a salt company in the 1920s, the list of uses include keeping the colors bright on boiled vegetables; making ice cream freeze; whipping cream rapidly; getting more heat out of boiled water; removing rust; sealing cracks; removing spots on clothes; putting out grease fires; killing poison ivy; and treating sprains, sore throats, and earaches. The salt industry goes still further, claiming 14,000 different uses for this under-appreciated substance!*
>
> *Until about a hundred years ago, when modern chemistry and geology revealed its prevalence, salt was one of the most sought after commodities. In times past, it has served as currency, been responsible for trade routes and the establishment of great cities, provoked and financed wars, and played a strategic part in others. Taxes on salt have secured empires and inspired revolution.*
>
> *The Romans appear to have esteemed salt highly. Its army, for a time, was even paid in salt. This is the origin of the word "salary" and the expressions "worth his salt" and "earning his salt." In fact, the Latin word sal became the French word solde, meaning "pay," and has come down to us in the word "soldier." The first of the great Roman roads was the Via Salaria, the Salt Road. The Romans used to salt their greens, which is the origin of the word "salad," salted.*
>
> *The movie Gandhi, portraying the life of Mohandas Gandhi, shows him choosing, as his means of rebellion against British colonialism, to*

contravene Britain's salt policy. Many of these and other historical tidbits can be found by reading *Salt, A World History* by Mark Kurlansky: a fascinating study of the only rock humans eat.

During the times in which the Bible was written, salt was much more precious, and people better understood its value. One use that is probably not on the salt industry's list is that salt was to accompany every offering. "And every offering of your grain offering you shall season with salt; you shall not allow the salt of the covenant of your God to be lacking from your grain offering. With all your offerings you shall offer salt" (Leviticus 2:13).

The altar symbolizes God's table. Since salt is always on our tables, God would have it always used at His, not to preserve the sacrifice but because it was the food of God's table and should be salted, especially the meat. It was so important that it was provided by the Temple (Ezra 7:20-22) and stored in a room, the Chamber of Salt, in the court of the Temple.

Notice the phrase "salt of the covenant" in Leviticus 2:13. It has been common throughout history for people to confirm their agreements with each other by eating and drinking together, at which times salt is used. As salt was added to foods, not only for spice but also to preserve them from decay, it became a symbol of incorruptibility and permanence. A "covenant of salt" signified an everlasting covenant, as we will see. In the Bible, salt also came to symbolize purity, perfection, wisdom, hospitality, durability, and fidelity.

The need for various animal sacrifices passed with the death of Jesus Christ. However, the apostle Paul urges us to "present [our] bodies a living sacrifice, holy, acceptable to God, which is [our] reasonable service" (Romans 12:1). The first eleven chapters of Romans are doctrinal in nature, and with Romans 12:1, Paul begins explaining the practical application of God's teaching. The first thing he mentions is that we are to be living sacrifices, holy and acceptable to God. For a sacrifice to be acceptable to God, it must be salted. So, in a symbolic manner, we must be salted as well...

AND GOD SAID:

Romans 12:1

Present [our] bodies a living sacrifice, holy, acceptable to God, which is [our] reasonable service.

AND GOD SAID:

Mark 9: 49-50

For everyone will be seasoned with fire, and every sacrifice will be seasoned with salt. Salt is good, but if the salt loses its flavor, how will you season it? Have salt in yourselves, and have peace with one another.

Salt Preserves

Prior to 1800, the only way to keep food for any length of time was to salt it. This method of food preservation declined when people discovered that they could seal food in jars and heat it, what is called "canning" today. Then, in 1809 in London, Peter Durand received a patent for preserving food in tin cans. Unfortunately, he failed to invent the can opener—that would not come for several more years.

Around this same time, people began to pack fish in ice. Packing other foods in ice was not practical, however, because, once the ice melted, the resulting water created an environment in which bacteria could flourish. An American inventor named Clarence Birdseye took care of this. During his life, he patented 250 inventions, but we remember him mostly for his method of freezing food.

Now, when we want something for dinner, we reach into our freezers for vegetables, meats, desserts, and the like. In earlier times, we would have gone to the storehouse and sliced off some salted meat, or to the cellar for pickled vegetables. Salt, therefore, has come to stand for durability, permanence, perpetuity, incorruptibility, and purity. This is why salt was used to ratify a covenant; it preserved and stood for permanence. In Numbers 18:19, God says to Aaron:

All the heave offerings of the holy things, which the children of Israel offer to the Lord, I have given to you and your sons and daughters with you as an ordinance forever; it is a covenant of salt forever before the Lord with you and your descendants with you.

Adam Clarke comments that "salt was the opposite of leaven, for it preserved from putrefaction and corruption, and signified the purity and persevering fidelity that were necessary in the worship of God."

The symbolism should be obvious to us as living sacrifices. We are to be without spot or blemish—pure, in other words. God does not change (Hebrews 13:8), and He does not lie (Numbers 23:19). He has made certain covenants with His people that cannot be broken. We have only to live a life of obedience, which God helps us to do. Our sacrifice, then, is not a one-time deal but is ongoing and perpetual. Salt preserves.

Salt Seasons

The New King James' heading above Mark 9:49 reads, "Tasteless Salt Is Worthless," which is certainly true. Most of us have probably never tasted salt that had lost its flavor, but we can easily understand the concept. Christ tells His disciples, "For everyone will be seasoned with fire, and every sacrifice will be seasoned with salt. Salt is good, but if the salt loses its flavor, how will you season it? Have salt in yourselves, and have peace with one another" (Mark 9:49-50).

This characteristic is somewhat the opposite of the first one. Obviously, sacrifices in the Old Testament were not salted to preserve them since the meat was consumed immediately. They were salted because it was the food of God's table, and no flesh is eaten without salt. Jesus says, "Every sacrifice will be seasoned with salt." Man is flesh, and his nature, corrupt (Genesis 6:3); therefore, his sacrifice must be seasoned and made more palatable.

Notice that Christ says, "Have salt in yourselves, and have peace with one another." How do we do this? The apostle Paul writes in Colossians 4:6, "Let your speech always be with grace, seasoned with salt, that you may know how you ought to answer each one." He is speaking specifically of answering those in the world, but should we not be even more gracious to those in our family?

The Greek word Paul uses, translated "grace," is charis, which means "graciousness, of manner or act, especially the divine influence upon the heart, and its reflection in the life." Matthew Henry's commentary says, "Grace is the salt which seasons our discourse, makes it savory and keeps it from corrupting."

The words that come from our mouths reflect upon us more than any other facet of our lives. When we gossip, are those words seasoned? Are they "savory" to the ears of others? When we speak in a hurtful manner to our family, both physical and spiritual, are those words seasoned?" (*14)

There is no question salt plays a significant role both physically and spiritually throughout scripture. Be it literal or metaphorical, salt heals, purifies, flavors, binds, and cleanses. Salt represents God's covenant with us through Christ; as a promise for truth and goodness.

AND GOD SAID:

Colossians 4: 6

Let your speech always be with grace, seasoned with salt, that you may know how you ought to answer each one.

Genesis 19: 26

But his wife looked back from behind him, and she became a pillar of salt.

Chapter Summary

Salt is a crucial substance our bodies need to be healthy and to function. The key, however, is to consume ONLY good salts and to avoid the unhealthy and toxic salts. Good salts are unrefined salts like Celtic Sea Salt, Himalayan Pink Salt, and Redmond's Real Salt. Toxic salts are refined salts like those found in almost all processed foods and standard table salt. Benefits of using unrefined salts are countless, a few of which include a balanced blood pressure, hydration, increased circulation, balanced blood sugar levels, better sleep, detoxification, and muscle tone. Spiritually, salt represents purity, fidelity, hospitality, and durability. A salt covenant represents an unbreakable bond, or promise.

Action Steps:

1. Take an inventory of what kind of salt you have currently in your spice cabinet and make sure you are only consuming an unrefined healthy variety as mentioned in this chapter.
2. Consider how much processed food you are consuming and replace these choices with living foods, whole foods, and healthier options to reduce the amount of unhealthy refined salt you are inadvertently consuming through these processed foods. This includes anything that comes in a box, can, or container with more than two or three pronounceable and recognizable ingredients.
3. Take a salt bath at least once a week, right before bed to assist your body with detoxing, de-stressing, and cleansing.

Notes:

Chapter 5: Bread of Life
(Grains, Legumes, Nuts, & Seeds)

Physical Significance of Grains, Legumes, Nuts, & Seeds

One of the most controversial topics in the health industry today is also one of the staple foods found in biblical times; gracing the pages of the Bible a whopping 492 times! What is this questionable food, why is it so controversial, and what do you need to know about it for your health? These questions, and more, will be addressed in this chapter; a chapter that is filled with enlightening information that will guide you in following God's guidelines on this topic, and will drastically change the health of many of you just by following a few simple changes. I'm referring to how we approach grains (and her cousins, Beans, Legumes, Nuts, and Seeds) in our diets.

Grains

Because grains are mentioned more often in the Bible than the other categories discussed in this chapter, we will start with grains, then share more insights about beans and legumes, nuts, and seeds. As you will see, most of the same rules apply once you understand a few basic, yet important concepts, particularly how best to prepare them for optimum nutrition and health.

"Grains" generally consist of a large family of edible seeds from specific grasses belonging to the botanical family "Poaceae", also known as Gramineae family. This includes wheat, barley, rye, rice, oats, kamut, spelt, teff, amaranth, sorghum, corn, quinoa, and buckwheat, to name a few.

During Biblical times, grains (particularly wheat and barley) were a staple part of their diets, often in the form of bread. Bread was so central on the Biblical table that the Hebrew word for "bread" also means "food". Grains were easily grown and cultivated, stored well, and were highly nourishing. In Exodus 9:31, we read that one of the plagues visited upon Pharaoh to convince him to let the Israelites leave Egypt was a rain of hailstones that ruined the grain fields. Grains were listed as one of the riches of the Promised Land that God held in store for the Israelites (Deuteronomy 8:8). Ruth arrived in Bethlehem with her mother-in-law, Naomi, at the beginning of the barley harvest and gleaned barley from the harvested fields (Ruth 1:22 and 2:17). Absalom destroyed Joab's grain fields to weaken his enemy (II Samuel 14:30). God instructed Ezekiel to make a bread with

AND GOD SAID:

Matthew 6: 11

Give us this day our daily bread.

Isaiah 55: 2

Why do you spend your money for that which is not bread, and your labor for that which does not satisfy? Listen diligently to me, and eat what is good, and delight yourselves in rich food. (ESV)

wheat, barley, beans, lentils, millet, and spelt (Ezekiel 4:9). And Jesus took five loaves of bread and fed 5,000 people, with such abundance that afterward his followers were able to collect twelve large baskets of leftover bread (John 6:1–13). (*22) These examples are just a few of the many times God's Word talks about this valuable and nourishing food that graced the tables during biblical times.

The bread of the Bible was much different than what we think of as bread today, however. The image we see in movies and church depictions of Jesus breaking a fluffy loaf of white bread during the last supper is not particularly accurate. In reality, most bread was made from just a few simple ingredients like flour, water, and salt. Flour was made by first sprouting and often fermenting the grains before grinding them into a powder using stones. This flour was made from the *sprouted whole grain*, not a refined or separated version of the grain, and the bread was made immediately after grinding.

Let's take a quick look at some of the major differences between what God considers healthy bread and what we have done to alter this perfect food, then discuss options that you can easily do to ensure your bread is following God's plan for your health.

First, we need to consider how the ingredients we are using to make our bread have changed. Modern bread is usually made from wheat that has been genetically modified, hybridized, and formulated to grow bigger, stronger, and faster with more pest resistance and more profitability. Structurally, modern wheat is much different than the wheat varieties more commonly grown during Biblical times. Studies conducted on modern wheat show some very interesting differences.

- Modern wheat has more gluten proteins which some specialists believe is contributing to the rise of gluten interferences, gluten intolerance, and gluten-related diseases.
- Modern wheat is lower in mineral content including zinc, magnesium, iron, copper, and selenium.
- Modern wheat contains more chromosomes (Einkorn, a variety that is considered an ancient wheat because it dates back over 5000 years, contains 14 chromosomes, whereas modern hard red wheat contains 46 chromosomes), which is believed to be a contributing factor in modern wheat being more difficult for the body to assimilate and digest.

- Modern wheat is a mutation caused by radiation, particularly in the form of gamma and microwave radiation to change the molecular structure of the grain making it less susceptible to disease, yet also more difficult for the body to digest.
- Modern wheat is grown with harmful pesticides including up to or exceeding 16 different pesticides. One of the common pesticides used on wheat is Malathion, found on over 50% of American wheat and is considered a "neurotoxin" which, when ingested, can affect our hormones and neurological systems. (*20)

We then take this new "better" wheat and process it so that all the life-force has been removed (since this is what will make the flour spoil or go rancid faster) creating a refined white flour that can easily be transported and stored for long periods of time. This refined white flour is then used to make our bread, cereals, pasta, crackers, cookies, and other grain products. However, even though the products made with this flour may taste good, there is little "light energy" found in the end product, very little nutrient value, and high levels of empty carbohydrate calories that convert to sugar in our system, contributing to weight gain, insulin imbalances, digestive upset, allergies, and inflammation in the body. Recent studies show that modern wheat, even the so-called healthier whole wheat, do several things in the body:

1. Modern hybridized wheat contains higher levels of proteins and more gluten that are both typically harder to digest. Gluten is a protein composite of gliadin and glutenin which give foods their delicious, chewy texture. Gluten also helps the dough keep its shape and it helps make a nice fluffy, light bread. According to Alessio Fasano, the Medical Director for the University of Maryland's Center for Celiac Research, gluten is very difficult for anyone to digest because we don't have the enzymes to break it down. (*21) Gliadin and Glutenin are considered "immunogenic anti-nutrients" which trigger systemic inflammation by the immune system which can lead to a number of illnesses including rheumatoid arthritis, IBS (irritable bowel syndrome), and celiac disease.
2. Modern wheat contains lectins which, when not cooked properly or when consumed in excess, can bind to insulin receptors and our intestinal lining, causing inflammation, contribute to autoimmune diseases, and insulin resistance.
3. Modern wheat contains phytic acid, which can't be digested by humans. Phytic acid also tends to bind itself to important minerals like calcium, magnesium, zinc, and iron, making them impossible for the body to absorb; consequently causing possible nutrient deficiencies which can lead to problems such as anemia and osteoporosis.

AND GOD SAID:

2 Corinthians 9:10

He who supplies seed to the sower and bread for food will supply and multiply your seed for sowing and increase the harvest of your righteousness. (ESV)

Genesis 18:5

While I bring a morsel of bread, that you may refresh yourselves, and after that you may pass on; since you have come to your servant.

4. Modern wheat has been linked to the body forming low-density lipoproteins (LDL) particles; which are responsible for atheroscelerotic plaque, which in turn can trigger heart disease and stroke. (*21)
5. Modern wheat feeds candida overgrowth, a harmful yeast that, when out of balance, can wreak havoc on the body causing a wide array of ailments including depression, brain fog, difficulty sleeping, and many other health problems including cancer.

It's no wonder that we're dealing with a health crisis today when you look at the effects modern wheat has on the body, coupled with the average American consuming over 133 pounds of wheat each year! (*23) Dr. William Davis, in his book "Wheat Belly", contributes our fascination and over-consumption of modern wheat to the common problem seen by many of us of that over-extended gut. In his book, Dr. Davis says:

A wheat belly represents the accumulation of fat that results from years of consuming foods that trigger insulin, the hormone fat storage. While some people store fat in their buttocks and thighs, most people collect ungainly fat around the middle. This 'central' or 'visceral' fat is unique: Unlike fat in other body areas, it provokes inflammatory phenomena, distorts insulin responses, and issues abnormal metabolic signals to the rest of the body...

...The consequences of [modern] wheat consumption, however, are not just manifested in the body's surface; wheat can also reach deep down into virtually every organ of the body, from the intestines, liver, heart, and thyroid gland all the way up to the brain. In fact, there's hardly an organ that is not affected by [modern] wheat in some potentially damaging way. (*29)

With so much science pointing out the detrimental effects of wheat, does that mean we have to give up wheat altogether? The good news is you don't necessarily have to give up wheat. You can still enjoy breads, pasta, pizza crusts, and all those delicious favorites that we have become accustomed to in our modern culture. We just have to make a few important changes to the *type* of wheat we choose and how we prepare it. God is clear in the Bible that wheat is healthy for us... as long as it is God's wheat and not the wheat that man has tried to make better.

As I mentioned before, Einkorn wheat is a variety of wheat that more closely resembles the wheat that was grown during Biblical times. It has not been modified, hybridized, or genetically changed. Studies show that Einkorn wheat is more digestible, contains more bio-available proteins, and has more minerals than other traditional wheat varieties. I have heard countless testimonials from people who switched to Einkorn and saw almost miraculous improvements in seasonal allergies, skin issues, digestive issues, and even neurological issues. Spelt and kamut are also ancient varieties of wheat that also are healthier alternatives to modern wheat.

Not an avid cook? That's ok, too! More and more we are seeing products like pasta and breads available on the market that have been made with ancient grains. If you can't find Einkorn, try switching to products made with quinoa, millet, or spelt. They are equally delicious and so much better for your body than modern wheat products.

Wheat is not the only grain, however. Prepared properly, being careful to choose ancient and organic varieties, all grains offer satisfying nourishment and delicious flavors. Wheat is the most common across the globe, yet other grains such as rice, quinoa, barley, spelt, teff, amaranth, corn, and buckwheat are wonderful too. Many of the other grains can be ground into flour and used in delicious recipes, such as rice flour, quinoa flour, and corn flour. Nut flours like almond flour and coconut flour can also often be substituted to make delicious and more healthy recipes.

Proper Preparation of Grains

Another thing to consider, other than the **type** of grain you are using is **how** you prepare the grains before using them in your recipes. Even most so-called "healthy" diets will tell you things like, "switch to whole grains" and "buy only organic". True, whole grains are better than refined... but keep in mind what we already discussed about the *type* of flour you are consuming... even if it is whole grain. Modern whole wheat should be completely avoided.

The other important piece of the equation that is often missed and overlooked, however, is that grains **must** be soaked and sprouted before consuming them for optimum digestion and absorption. Grains in the Bible were almost always soaked and often fermented prior to consumption or making into recipes. Why is this important? Great question! Grains, in essence, are tiny embryos of baby plants that were designed by God to create a new life in the form of another plant. Each tiny grain seed contains all the nutrients, DNA, and energy needed to grow into a

Acts 2: 46

AND GOD SAID:

And day by day, attending the temple together and breaking bread in their homes, they received their food with glad and generous hearts.

Genesis 27: 17

And she put the delicious food and the bread, which she had prepared, into the hand of her son. (ESV)

stalk of grass that could produce more grain seeds, should that grain seed be planted. In order to protect the grain during this time until it is ready to grow, God gave that seed a protective barrier that surrounds the nutrient-dense inner part of the seed. That protective barrier is called an enzyme inhibitor; which serves two purposes. The first purpose is to slow down the inner enzymes of the seed so it is ready to grow when the conditions are ideal. The second purpose is to protect the seed from predators, because those enzyme inhibitors are toxic.

When we grind grains into flour when the grain is in its dormant state, those enzyme inhibitors are still present in the flour. This is why some people, who are more sensitive to the toxins created by those enzyme inhibitors, have serious reactions to grain products. Others, who may not be so sensitive, still experience reactions. They just may not be quite so obvious; or are attributed to normal life, such as allergies, inflammation, bloating, digestive upsets, gas, skin issues, and sleep issues. Over time, these reactions can compound into chronic disorders and diseases.

Think of it this way. Animals who are grain eaters generally have multiple stomachs (ruminants) like cattle, goats, sheep, deer, and camels. When these animals eat grains, the grain and forage mix with saliva, then move through the various stomachs, mixing with bacteria, then back into the mouth for further chewing (cud) before working its way through the entire digestion process. As a result, they can break through these enzyme inhibitors and maximize the nutrition found in the grain. Horses, rabbits, and pigs only have one stomach like we do. Feed them too much grain and it can kill them, particularly horses who have small stomachs and large intestines, relative to their size.

The good news is that we can easily neutralize the enzyme inhibitors before consuming grain products. All we have to do is sprout the grains first! Sprouting is simply soaking the grains in water for a short period of time to "trick" the grains into thinking it is time to grow. At this point, the enzyme inhibitor is expelled and the inner hydrolytic (water activated) enzymes become activated. The coolest part, though, is that not only do we no longer need to worry about the toxicity of the enzyme inhibitors, but the grain is now no longer dormant, making them even more nutritious.

Grains consist of three parts: the germ, the endosperm, and the bran. The germ is the plant embryo and contains all the DNA of the plant. The endosperm is the starchy portion that feeds the embryo during growth until the plant can sustain itself from photosynthesis in its leaves. The bran is the outer part of the grain that provides some nutrients and also provides protection to the germ. When the grain sprouts, the life-force of the grain is activated and the best part is that the hydrolytic enzymes convert the endosperm from long-term-storage starches into simpler molecules that are easily digested by the plant embryo. As a result, the grain is much easier for us to digest, too, and has higher levels of bio-available nutrients like B vitamins, vitamin C, folate, fiber, minerals, and essential amino acids like lysine. (*24)

Commercially, you can find sprouted whole grains and sprouted flour. Or, you can make your own by purchasing whole grain, soaking it for 8-12 hours, then draining the water from the grains. Rinse and drain again after another 12 hours and repeat until a small "tail" appears on the grain.

Sprouted grains can be used in two ways:
- Wet Method: After sprouting, the grains are still somewhat "wet" from the moisture used to sprout them. At this point, you can mash them or grind them using a food processor into a thick puree to make breads, tortillas, or muffins. In some cases, you can also just consume the whole sprouted grain in recipes as is, without grinding or mashing them, such as porridge recipes.
- Dry Method: After sprouting, the grains are dried in a dehydrator on a low setting to maintain the nutrient content in the grain. Once dry, the grains can be stored for a short time (a couple weeks) or ground into flour using a grain mill to make sprouted whole grain flour, which then can be made into any of your favorite recipes including bread, muffins, pancakes, cookies, crackers, cakes, pizza crusts, etc.

Making the switch to sprouted ancient grains could be one of the most valuable changes you can make for your health. In our home, we went completely off of wheat altogether for a period of time to help reset our digestive system and eliminate a candida overgrowth (harmful yeast). We then made the switch to sprouted Einkorn wheat for baking and recipes and the difference was and is amazing. I have found that when I eat modern wheat, such as at a restaurant or at a friend's house, my skin starts to crack again, I get bloated, and my allergies return. For bread, we love using sprouted Einkorn flour with a sourdough starter to make a truly delicious and filling sourdough bread.

Sourdough is a method of leavening bread using natural bacteria and yeasts rather than a commercial fast-acting yeast. Because the process of making sourdough

AND GOD SAID:

Ezekiel 4: 9

But as for you, take wheat, barley, beans, lentils, millet, and spelt, and put them into one vessel and make them into bread for yourself. (AMP)

AND GOD SAID:

2 Samuel 17: 28-29

David brought beds, basins, pottery, wheat, flour, parched grain, broad
beans, lentils, honey cream, and cheese of the herd...to eat. (AMP)

bread requires more proofing time in which the natural yeasts are breaking down
the gluten in the bread, most sourdough breads are more digestible than yeast
breads. A good sprouted-grain sourdough bread, made from ancient grains like
Einkorn wheat, is the closest we will get in modern times to the bread mentioned
in the bible. Best of all, it is incredibly delicious and satisfying!

Ezekiel Bread

Probably the most famous bread recipe found in the Bible is in the book of Ezekiel
when God instructed to "take wheat and barley, beans and lentils, millet and
spelt, and put them into a single vessel and bake your bread from them" (Ezekiel
4:9). God gave this recipe to the Israelites to help them get through the
upcoming 390 days of exile they were about to face. Interestingly, when you
combine the ingredients God gave us in this verse, you get a complete protein,
with all the essential amino acids needed to sustain life. Granted, the bread is
very dense, hearty, and filling as it was designed to support life during a time of
famine. Ezekiel bread is also made solely from sprouted grains and legumes.

Although personally I enjoy the occasional Ezekiel bread in my diet, it is
important to remember the context in which this verse was written. God was
giving his people a survivalist fare that they would be eating as a result of their
sinful ways. Basically, He was saying that as a result of your sin, THIS is what
you will be reduced to eating... and for over a year because you haven't repented
of your sins!

Should you want to try it for yourself, you can find commercially distributed
loaves of Ezekiel bread, in various flavors, at most local health food stores or
grocers, and these loaves are quite tasty. Keep in mind, however, that the
commercial loaves will still be made using modern wheat as one of the
ingredients, so I wouldn't recommend it if you have an illness you are trying to
heal from or if you have a wheat sensitivity. My daughter especially likes the
cinnamon raison version of this commercial variety, but we save it for special
occasions or when traveling.

You can also make your own, yet this recipe is not what I would recommend for
the beginner cook as it can be a bit tricky and temperamental, and the resulting
loaf is very different from what most of us are accustomed to in our bread.

Beans and Legumes

"Beans and Legumes" generally consist of edible seeds from plants in the botanical family "Fabaceae", also known as Leguminosae family. In the Bible, these foods are sometimes referred to as "pulse". Beans (which are actually legumes) include all dry beans such as black beans, kidney beans, northern white beans, adzuki beans, mung beans, navy beans, pinto beans, lima beans, and butter beans. Legumes includes examples such as chickpeas, lentils, soybeans, edamame, cowpeas, black-eyed peas, carob, peanuts, tamarind, lupins, and others.

Beans and legumes are, in my opinion, some of the most unsung heroes in the food world. Extremely economical to stock and prepare, these amazing foods are excellent sources of protein, fiber, folate, B vitamins, iron, zinc, magnesium, and potassium. They are low in calories and high in complex carbohydrates which generally means they are very filling.

The Story of Daniel

The book of Daniel contains fascinating and powerful stories of faith, courage, and nutrition. More than any other book of the Bible, Daniel gives us great insight into what God desires for us and what can be achieved through faith, a close relationship with God, and adherence to his rules on diet. As a first-hand account, written by Daniel himself, we learn of how King Nebuchadnezzar conquers Judah and takes the very best of the best from Judah's people back to Babylon. Only the most handsome, wise, and skillful men and women were chosen, including Daniel and his three friends Hananiah, Mishael, and Azariah. Daniel and his friends were then given Babylonian names. Daniel became known as Belteshazzar. Hananiah was named Shadrach, Mishael became Meshach, and Azariah became Abed-nego.

Daniel and his friends were not prisoners of war, but more like honored guests and King Nebuchanadnezzer ordered only the finest wine and richest food to be served to them. It is unclear exactly what this food entailed, but Daniel does tell us that he would not "defile, taint, or dishonor himself with the king's finest food; so he asked the commander of the officials that he might be excused" (Daniel 1: 8) and to be allowed to eat what was healthy. As the story goes, he offered a test; to be allowed 10 days to eat as he wanted and if after that time he didn't prove that his way was better, then he would eat what they wanted him to. According to Daniel 1: 12, Daniel and his friends ate only water, pulses, and vegetables for those 10 days.

AND GOD SAID:

Genesis 25: 34

Then Jacob gave Esau bread and lentil stew; and he ate and drank, and got up and went on his way. In this way Esau scorned his birthright. (AMP)

AND GOD SAID:

Genesis 43: 11

Then their father Israel said to them, "If it must be, then do this: Put some of the best products of the land in your bags and take them down to the man as a gift--a little balm and a little honey, some spices and myrrh,

After the trial period, all were amazed to see that not only did Daniel and his friends thrive on their fare of water, pulses, and vegetables...but they were ten times better than all the advisors, teachers, magicians, or scholars of the whole realm. (Daniel 1: 20)

As we mentioned earlier, pulses are another name for legumes and beans, particularly sprouted legumes. With their high protein content, complex carbohydrates, and myriad of vitamins and minerals, it is no surprise that Daniel and his friends thrived on this simple diet consisting primarily of sprouted beans and legumes.

Proper Preparation of Beans and Legumes

When consuming beans and legumes, however, it is important to recognize that they are essentially seeds and follow the same principles for proper preparation as grains. Most dry beans and legumes contain enzyme inhibitors, making them difficult to digest. These enzyme inhibitors contribute to the common problem of gas and bloating after consuming.

As with grains, we can easily bypass this challenge by simply soaking and/or sprouting them first. Soaking dry beans before cooking releases the enzyme inhibitors, softens the hard outer shell, and increases the bio-available nutrients. Soaking and sprouting beans such as adzuki beans and mung beans make a power-packed, protein-rich raw snack that can be eaten straight or added to salads, soups, smoothies, snack mixes, and granola. Spouted lentils are delicious as a raw snack or lightly cooked in a wide variety of soups, stews, and side-dish recipes. Sprouted peas are exceptionally sweet and are one of our favorites for eating raw, adding to salads, and including in recipes.

Beans and legumes can also be ground into flour. Any recipe that calls for regular flour can be altered to include up to 25% bean flour, which adds the additional protein and nutrients found in the beans. For example, in a muffin recipe that calls for 2 cups flour, you could use 1 ½ cups sprouted Einkorn flour and ½ cup bean flour instead. If makiing your own bean flour, try soaking and sprouting the beans first then dehydrating them before grinding into flour. Never use kidney beans for bean flour as kidney beans can be toxic if not properly soaked and cooked.

Bean flour can also be used as a thickening agent instead of corn starch in soups and gravies. For every cup of soup stock, water, or bouillon, combine 3-4 tablespoons of bean, pea, or lentil flour in a small amount of cool water. Stir with a whisk to thoroughly combine and remove any lumps. Slowly stir the combination into boiling stock and whisk briskly until thickened to desired consistency. We often use bean flour to make our own healthier versions of cream of mushroom soup, cream of celery soup, and cream of chicken soup. We've included our recipes in the Recipe Section, later in this book.

I encourage you to experiment with beans and lentils and discover for yourself the endless bounty of flavors they add to your meals. And the best part is that you can enjoy this hearty and filling fare while knowing you are adding nourishment that truly supports health and wellness, according to God's design.

Nuts

Generally speaking, when we are talking about nuts in culinary terms, we are referring to any oily kernels found within a shell and used for food. This includes examples such as almonds, Brazil nuts, cashews, chestnuts, hazelnuts, Macadamia nuts, pecans, pine nuts, pistachios, and walnuts. Although coconut is technically a fruit, other characteristics for cooking and eating more closely resemble nuts, so we are also including coconut in this category.

Nuts are not commonly mentioned in the Bible, but there are enough references that allude to nuts being a regular part of the biblical diet, particularly almonds, pistachios, and walnuts. Nuts are considered to be a good source of healthy fats, vitamin E, vitamin B2, folate, fiber, magnesium, phosphorus, potassium, copper, selenium, and essential amino acids.

Nuts, like grains and legumes, will contain enzyme inhibitors and are best consumed after soaking the raw nut. The enzyme inhibitors on nuts are particularly difficult to digest, making soaking especially important. Commercially, nuts are often purchased as already roasted, salted, and flavored. I generally recommend avoiding these nuts since it is highly unlikely that the manufacturer properly soaked and dried the nuts before roasting. Without this step, however, nuts are difficult to digest and can cause inflammation in the body; which is one explanation for the rise of nut allergies we are seeing, especially in our kids.

AND GOD SAID:

1 Corinthians 11: 23-24

The Lord Jesus, on the night he was betrayed, took bread, and when he had given thanks, he broke it and said, "This is my body, which is for you; do this in remembrance of me. (NIV)

Deuteronomy 8:3

Man does not live by bread alone, but man lives by every word that proceeds out of the mouth of the Lord. (AMP)

Properly prepared nuts make wonderful snacks, delicious additions to recipes, and fantastic flour substitutes when soaked, dried, and ground. Almond flour and coconut flour, in particular, are family favorites for muffins, cookies, and pie crusts. To properly prepare nuts, purchase raw nuts in quantities that fit your rate of consumption. The oils in nuts can go rancid quickly, so they are best consumed as fresh as possible. Store unused nuts in the freezer until you are ready to soak them and enjoy them, to keep the nuts fresh for a longer period of time. Soak raw nuts in fresh water (not chlorinated or treated water) for 8-12 hours. Drain, rinse, and drain again. Dry on a dehydrator to make them crunchy again, or use immediately for recipes using soft nuts, like nut butters and nut milks. An exception to this rule is coconut, as it is actually a fruit and the meat of the coconut that we are consuming does not contain enzyme inhibitors.

Seeds

In addition to the grains, beans, legumes, and nuts that we have mentioned are other seeds that are loaded with delicious goodness while contributing to a healthy diet. These seeds include examples like chia seeds, flax seeds, sesame seeds, hemp seeds, sunflower seeds, and pumpkin seeds.

Small seeds such as these generally don't release as much toxicity in their enzyme inhibitors and can be consumed without soaking them; although soaking and sprouting is certainly acceptable. Seeds are excellent sources of fiber, healthy fats, omega fatty acids, vitamins, trace minerals, and phytonutrients.

Spiritual Significance of Grains

With grains making up a significant portion of the basic biblical diet, it is no surprise that grains share a symbolic significance throughout scripture. In the Old Testament, grains were used to represent God's presence (Exodus 25:30), hospitality (Genesis 19:3), and the acceptance of wisdom (Proverbs 9:5). In the New Testament, grains (bread in particular), symbolized Jesus and the eternal life he offers to those willing to follow him (John 6:32-35, 41, 50-51).

John 6:51 (NIV) says, "I am the living bread that came down from heaven. If anyone eats of this bread, he will live forever. This bread is my flesh, which I will give for the life of the world."

"Jesus came to earth and announced, "I am the living, bread that came down from Heaven." Through Christ Jesus, a whole new dimension of living has been made available to us. When we accept Jesus Christ into our heart and life, partaking by faith in His broken body and shed blood, we walk into a new dimension of life.

Natural bread is earthly, but spiritual bread is heavenly. Natural bread is corruptible, but spiritual bread is incorruptible. Natural bread is limited, but spiritual bread is unlimited. Natural bread feeds the body; spiritual bread feeds the spirit." (*26)

Scripture mentions two different kinds of bread: leavened and unleavened. Leavened bread was made using fermentation or some form of "cultures" to get the bread to rise; much like modern sourdough breads. The discovery of "yeast" for breads didn't arrive on the scene until much later in history. In many cases, leavened bread represented corruption and sin, such as 1 Corinthians 5:8 when Paul mentions "the leaven of malice and wickedness."

Unleavened bread represents Christ, in his abounding love for us, and the spiritual fulfillment and nourishment that He offers. It is through Jesus that our spiritual bodies are truly fed. In most cases when we read about bread in the Bible, it is used to represent "that which is taken into the body and provides nourishment." (*27) In the Lord's Prayer, when we beseech God to "give us this day our daily bread," we are not only asking that our physical nourishment needs are met; but also that God fill our hearts and our spirits with His presence each day. God does not live in us uninvited, rather He gives us free will to choose to have a relationship with Him.

"In the Bible, bread is provision, it is blessing, it is strength. It is the product of dominion, a cooperation between God's blessing on the crops and man's labor in the fields, the mill and the bakery. Every loaf of bread is God's kindness, a demonstration of the image of God, of God's will being done on earth as it is in heaven, and when we eat this blessing, we receive strength." (*28)

Have you ever finished a meal and still felt hungry; like something was missing? Unsatisfied? You find yourself craving something more, but not sure what? It may not be that you're physically hungry; rather you may be spiritually hungry. The emptiness you feel can only be filled by feeding on the Word, turning to God,

AND GOD SAID:

John 6: 36

I am the bread of life. He who comes to me will never go hungry, and he who believes in me will never be thirsty. (NIV)

and welcoming Him into your life, your day, and your situation. And, spiritual fulfillment is so much more satisfying than any of the greatest, most deliciously prepared meal you have ever experienced; a fulfillment that only comes from God.

Chapter Summary:

Grains, beans, legumes, nuts, and seeds play an important role both in our physical health and spiritual well-being. Physically, these powerful foods contain building blocks for life in the form of carbohydrates, proteins, fats, vitamins, minerals, amino acids, phytonutrients, omegas, and enzymes. The key to unlocking the power of these foods, however, is by first choosing varieties that are closest to what God created, not what Man created and grown in a way that supports God's creation. Then, we need to prepare them properly by soaking (and sometimes sprouting) them to release the enzyme inhibitors and increase nutritional value.

Spiritually, "grain" and "bread" has great meaning, particularly as Jesus himself being the "Bread of Life." Jesus is where we get our spiritual sustenance and it is only through Him that we may never again be spiritually hungry.

Action Steps:

1. Reduce (or better yet, eliminate) processed wheat from your diet. Replace with healthier grain or nut choices that have been properly prepared by soaking first. Breads, pasta, cookies, crackers, etc. should be from ancient soaked grains only.
2. Add some form of soaked beans, soaked legumes, soaked nuts, and seeds into your diet every day. This gives variety, nutrients, flavor, and energy to your culinary routine.
3. The next time you take communion, prayerfully and deeply consider the significant symbolism of what the bread represents and how partaking of this last supper impacts your life and your spiritual walk.

Theologenic Diet
Grains, Beans, Legumes, and Seeds

The following is a summary of foods you can enjoy, and suggested preparation as discussed in this chapter. This list is by no means complete as there are thousands of varieties available, yet is meant as a basic guideline to get you started and show you the diversity of healthy options available.

Grains:

Einkorn Wheat (sprouted, flour)
Oats (sprouted, flour, rolled)
Rye (sprouted, flour)
Spelt (sprouted, flour)
Kamut (flour)
Rice: Brown, Black, or Wild (soaked, flour,
        cooked)
Corn: look for non-GMO varieties (sprouted, flour, cooked)
Popcorn (popped)
Quinoa (sprouted, flour, cooked)
Barley (sprouted, cooked)
Amaranth (sprouted, flour, cooked)
Buckwheat (sprouted, cooked)

Beans:

Note: we don't recommend commercially canned beans since they have high amounts of unhealthy salts and haven't generally been processed correctly for optimum health and nutrition).

Kidney beans (soaked and cooked)
Black beans (soaked and cooked)
White Northern beans (soaked and cooked)
Cannelloni beans (soaked and cooked)
Pinto beans (soaked and cooked)
Navy beans (soaked and cooked)
Lima beans (soaked and cooked)
Garbanzo beans/Chickpeas (sprouted)
Mung beans (sprouted)
Adzuki beans (sprouted)

Legumes:

Peas (raw, sprouted, shoots, cooked)
Lentils (sprouted, cooked)
Edamame (raw, cooked)
Cowpeas (soaked, sprouted, cooked)
Black-eyed peas (soaked, sprouted, cooked)

Nuts:

Note: For best results, purchase raw organic nuts rather than commercially prepared or flavored nuts.

Almonds (soaked, raw, flour, milk, butter)
Brazil nuts (soaked)
Cashew (raw, roasted, milk, butter)
Chestnuts (soaked, roasted)
Hazelnuts (soaked, butter)
Macadamia nuts (soaked, roasted)
Pecans (soaked, raw, roasted, flour, butter)
Pine nuts (soaked, roasted)
Pistachios (soaked, raw, roasted)
Walnuts (soaked, raw, roasted)

Seeds:

Chia seeds (soaked, smoothies, ground)
Flax seeds (sprouted, ground)
Sesame seeds (sprouted, toasted, roasted)
Hemp seeds (raw)
Sunflower seeds (raw, sprouted, shoots)
Pumpkin seeds (raw, sprouted,

Notes:

Chapter 6: Garden of Eden (Vegetables, Fruits, & Greens)

Physical Significance of Vegetables, Fruits, & Greens

From the beginning of time when God first created man in the Garden of Eden, the foundation of our diet was vegetables, fruits, greens, herbs, nuts, and seeds. And despite all the controversy in fad diets on things like fats, proteins, and carbohydrates; one of the few things most diets will agree upon is the importance of consuming lots of fresh vegetables, fruits, and greens. Having grown up on a small farm with a sizable vegetable garden, orchard, and berry patch, I was blessed to get to enjoy fresh produce from an early age. As a small child, the garden was a fun place to play; enjoying the colors, sounds, and smells of life... listening to buzzing bees alighting on blooms from cucumbers, squash, and peppers while delightfully snacking on fresh peas and cherry tomatoes; the feel of the soft dirt between my bare toes while I hid in the shade of the towering sweet corn stalks. Each season had its own bounty of colors and flavors, nourishing the body yet delighting the soul.

My appreciation for the family garden grew as I got older, particularly after the birth of my daughter. For the first time in my life, I was completely responsible for the well-being of an innocent and beautiful life who looked to me in total trust for her care. Deep in my spirit, through an indescribable love, I wanted to do all I could to give her the very best; so she could be healthy, happy, and fulfilled. In my mind, the logical place to turn was the garden. Some of her first solid foods came from what we were able to grow, and to this day she is an avid fan of a wide variety of vegetables, fruits, and greens; often choosing them over less healthy options. Even at just months old, she would spend time with me in the garden, and as she got older we often enjoyed spending time together planting seeds, tending plants, pulling weeds, and harvesting all the fruits of our efforts. In fact, we still do!

After my husband was diagnosed with a rare form of cancer at the base of his skull, the garden became not only a form of supplementing our grocery budget, but a crucial part of his treatment and recovery process. Before that, eating healthier was more of a "guideline" and a hobby rather than a lifestyle. Making

AND GOD SAID:

Genesis 1: 29

And God said, behold, I have given you every herb bearing seed, which is upon the face of all the earth, and every tree, in which is the fruit of a tree yielding seed; to you it shall be for food. (KJV)

Daniel 1: 16

So the steward took away their food and the wine they were to drink, and gave them vegetables. (ESV)

the commitment to do what needed to be done and eat according to God's plan was no longer something we could take lightly. The cornerstone of his healing from within came from the delightful colors and varying textures of so many wonderful fresh, organic, and in-season living foods. No other collective group of foods on the planet offer as much for our health than those found in the plant kingdom. Unfortunately, too often we wait until we are faced with a life-threatening illness before we are willing to make adjustments to our lifestyle and follow God's plan. Don't wait until it's too late for you and your loved ones!

Let's take a closer look at why vegetables, fruits, and greens were part of God's original diet, given to us through God's generosity and love, how they impact our health, and how best to enjoy them.

Nutrient Density

It should come as no surprise that vegetables, fruits, and greens are good for you and an important part of any diet; yet understanding *why* they are so good for you may be new information. As discussed in Chapter 1, the foundation to all life is energy; and energy on earth comes from the sun. Plants capture the sun's energy, and through photosynthesis they convert that energy and store it in the cells of the leaves, stems, roots, fruits, and flowers. When we eat vegetables, fruits, and greens, we are consuming "light energy" that our bodies need to heal and to thrive.

Breaking it down further, vegetables, fruits, and greens contain concentrated amounts of vital components needed for health including vitamins, minerals, enzymes, complex carbohydrates, fiber, amino acids, protein, and phytonutrients.

Phytonutrients

Phytonutrients, also sometimes referred to as phytochemicals, are chemicals produced by plants to perform various functions within the plant to stay healthy. Interestingly, these functions also help *our* bodies stay healthy. Phytonutrients also give plants, fruits, and vegetables their color through the pigmentations. Generally, the deeper the color, the richer the phytonutrients. It is often the intensity of phytonutrients that make some foods "superfoods" with powerful benefits to health. Consuming phytonutrients through vegetables, fruits, and greens offer a wide range of benefits to the body. Phytonutrients can reduce inflammation in the body, repair DNA damage, enhance immunity, support intercellular communication, detoxify cells, and balance metabolism. (*30)

The deep implication of phytonutrients and their impact on health are still not fully understood, partly due to their scope and complexity. For example, an apple contains upwards of 10,000 different phytonutrients all working symbiotically and synonymously together, of which cannot be duplicated or replicated in a lab through synthetic foods. What I mean is, you can't take any man-made supplement or vitamin that can give you the same benefits as a real apple, particularly when consumed fresh. This same rule applies with all the fruits, vegetables, and greens.

Since there are more than 25,000 identified phytonutrients, all of which are beneficial to our health, it is recommended to eat a wide variety of vegetables, fruits, and greens in as many colors as you can each day. Not only do the colors add a wide range of nutrient density to your food, but it also adds visual variety and appeal.

With so many different discovered phytonutrients, science has divided them into defined "classes" and "groups" for easier identification and study. Breaking things down even further to give you greater perspective, let's take a quick look at a couple phytonutrient categories that scientists consider particularly beneficial. For the sake of time, space, and not boring you with a textbook-worth of scientific information, I'll just go over a few of my favorites which are particularly noteworthy.

1. *Chlorophyll:* Chlorophyll is the most commonly known class of phytonutrients and is the phytochemical which gives leaves their green color. Benefits of consuming chlorophyll are numerous. For example, chlorophyll has the amazing ability to help increase the production of red blood cells, because the chemical structure closely resembles hemoglobin. In fact, during World War II, when doctors ran out of available blood for transfusions and surgeries on the field, they used a form of liquid chlorophyll instead with excellent results! Chlorophyll also has anti-inflammatory properties, increase oxygen to the cells, kills some strains of pathogenic yeasts, rejuvenates cells, reduces body odor, and helps control food cravings. (*31) Chlorophyll also helps the body with detoxification, which is particularly beneficial in our modern world of constant exposure to various toxins. Some of the best sources of chlorophyll are from consuming foods like dark leafy greens (such as collards, chard, kale,

AND GOD SAID:

Numbers 11:5

We remember the fish which we used to eat free in Egypt, the cucumbers and the melons and the leeks and the onions and the garlic...

AND GOD SAID:

Proverbs 15: 17

Better is a dish of vegetables where love is than a fattened ox served with hatred.

spinach), grasses (such as wheatgrass or barley grass), and microgreens (such as sunflower, kale, cabbage, and radish greens... I'll discuss microgreens in greater detail later in this chapter).

2. *Caratenoids:* Scientists have identified over 600 different phytonutrients in the caratenoid classification, most of which help plants, leaves, fruits, and vegetables develop their deep orange, yellow, and red colors. Caratenoids are beneficial for their antioxidant activity, contributions to eye health, immune system support, intercellular communication, and reduced risk of cancer and cardiovascular disease, according to the Linus Pauling Institute (*30). Caratenoids can be found in vegetables and fruits such as spinach, kale, carrots, pumpkins, yams, sweet potatoes, tomatoes, bell peppers, papaya, watermelon, cantaloupe, mangos, and oranges. Interestingly, in order for the body to properly absorb caratenoids and get the most benefit, all caratenoids must be consumed with a fat. I'll talk more about what constitutes healthy fats in Chapter 8, but suffice it to say that you should enjoy your caratenoid fruits and vegetables with some good organic butter, olive oil, or other healthy fat!

3. *Curcumin:* Curcumin is a phytonutrient that is most commonly found in root herbs like turmeric and ginger. This powerful phytonutrient with a distinctive deep yellow color has been getting more media attention lately due to its amazing ability to reduce pain and inflammation. Curcumin also reduces oxidative stress from free radicals, detoxifies, lowers bad (LDL) cholesterol, increases good (HDL) cholesterol, and has been effective in some clinical trials with combating cancer cell growth. (*30)

4. *Flavonoids:* Flavonoids are a very diverse group of phytonutrients and are found across a large range of foods such as apples, onions, coffee, grapefruit, tea, berries, chocolate, legumes, red wine, broccoli, cabbage, kale, leeks, tomatoes, ginger, lemons, parsley, carrots and buckwheat to name just a few. (*30) The primary benefit of flavonoids are their ability to support health and longevity, reduce the risk of cardiovascular disease, and cancers. Most likely, all those health-related articles, blogs, or reports you may have read extolling the health benefits of a certain food were most likely referring to the flavonoids in them. Not to be mistaken for an all-access pass to consume too much chocolate or wine because it's "good for you", it is important to understand the underlying reason why these reports tout certain foods as being healthy; namely, in particular, the phytonutrients they possess.

5. *Anthocyanins:* Anthocyanins are the phytonutrients that give vegetables, fruits, and greens their red, purple, and blue coloring such as those found

in red cabbage, red onions, kidney beans, elderberries, red or purple grapes, blueberries, acai berries, goji berries, bilberries, raspberries, black currants, strawberries, cherries, pomegranates, and red tomatoes. High in antioxidants and found to be anti-inflammatory, anti-viral, and anti-cancer, anthocyanins have been used in holistic medicine for thousands of years to treat cardiovascular issues, cancers, cognitive issues, and even the common cold as anthocyanins are known to boost the immune system and support cellular health.

It seems like every time I look on social media or read information about nutrition, I see another article about how certain vegetables, fruits, or greens can improve health. "New research shows....", "Avocados are good for the heart...", "Carrots help with the eyes..." These articles imply that just by eating carrots, your vision will be improved. Where it is true that the phytonutrients in carrots support the eyes (among other things), it is the collective result of the diet and lifestyle as a whole, with a wide diversity of phytonutrients, vitamins, minerals, enzymes, and amino acids found in your food, working together, that has the biggest impact on your health. The next time you read one of these articles, recognize the power of phytonutrients and how adding as many of them to your diet each day will greatly support all major functions of your body.

Interestingly, phytonutrients are not found in any other food source other than plant-based whole foods, particularly in their living or freshest state. This again takes us back to the awesome wonders of God's creations and how intricate life is...yet also so simple. The more "light energy" we consume, the more "life energy" we will receive.

Microgreens

Microgreens are one of the most powerful superfoods on the planet, and unfortunately these delicious powerhouses are little known and seldom included in daily dietary routines. When a seed is germinated and starts to grow from its dormant status, the seed releases the enzyme inhibitors (as mentioned in the previous chapter on grains), increases the bio-available nutrients, and starts to grow. The first stage of the seed growth is the "sprout" stage, which is identified when the seed swells, then starts to grow its first "root", visually identified by a small "tail" coming from the seed. In some cases, sprouts in and of themselves are a delicious addition to your dietary routine. Some of our family's favorite sprouts include Mung bean sprouts, Adzuki bean sprouts, garbanzo bean sprouts, sunflower sprouts, pea sprouts, and lentil sprouts to name a few.

AND GOD SAID:

Genesis 1:30

And to every beast of the earth and to every bird of the sky and to every thing that moves on the earth which has life, I have given every green plant for food. (AMV)

Deuteronomy 11: 10

For the land which you go in to possess is not like the land of Egypt, from which you came out, where you sowed your seed and watered it with your foot laboriously as in a garden of vegetables.

After a short period of time, the seed continues to grow and the first stem and cotyledon (first set of leaves) develops. At this point, the baby plant is now at the microgreens stage and can be harvested and enjoyed in various recipes, added to soups, salads, juices, and smoothies, or just eaten raw. Some of our family's favorite microgreens include sunflower greens, pea shoots, green cabbage, red cabbage, kale, broccoli, radish, lettuce, cilantro, dill, parsley, alfalfa, and radish greens to name a few.

Not only do microgreens taste amazing, with a much more potent flavor than their adult counterparts, microgreens tend to pack a powerful nutrient punch. In most cases, microgreens contain upwards of 7-70 times the vitamins, minerals, enzymes, and phytonutrients than their adult versions! Consuming microgreens is almost like taking a living supplement that tastes great and is super economical, easy to grow yourself even if you don't have a garden, and takes only about a week from the time you plant the seeds until you harvest and enjoy!

If you're not familiar with microgreens, I recommend you give them a try. If you are already enjoying microgreens from time to time, I encourage you to increase the amount and frequency with which you enjoy them.

Kids love microgreens, too! My daughter especially loves kale microgreens. We grow them year-round, indoors, in trays in the kitchen. Recently, I went to water a tray of kale microgreens and she had written in her characteristic artistic handwriting on a blue sticky note and stuck it on the side of the tray. The note read, "Megan's Kale! Mine. Nom-nom!" At first, my family and friends would lovingly tease me about becoming a rabbit the way I was eating, and that's ok. I knew that most of their light-hearted ribbing was in part due to a misguided cultural paradigm, created from years of brilliant, targeted marketing. It is our responsibility to become more informed, and to consider God's plan for our lives, even if it may seem "weird" at first.

I could write an entire book just about microgreens including how to grow them, nutrient value, and my favorite ways to eat them. For the sake of keeping this book from exceeding the length of the Bible with all that could be said about each topic, I will restrain myself for now and share with you the basics. If you are interested in learning more (which I highly encourage), I have created an entire online course to teach you all you would need to know to get started. Specific information on where you can find this information is included in our "Resources" section.

Sea Vegetables (Seaweed)

Another unsung hero in the health-food world that warrants some special attention includes sea vegetables or ocean vegetables. Sea vegetables include seaweeds such as nori (used for sushi), kelp, dulse, wakame, arame, kombu, agar agar, and hijiki, (to name a few) and are powerful sources of nutrients and "life energy".

Sea vegetables are particularly noteworthy "because they offer one of the broadest ranges of minerals of any food, containing virtually all the minerals found in the ocean—and not surprisingly, many of same minerals found in human blood. They also offer a variety of unique phytonutrients, including their sulfated polysaccharides (also called fucoidans)...Sea vegetables are an excellent source of iodine, vitamin C, manganese, and vitamin B2. They are also a very good source of vitamin A (in the form of carotenoids) and copper as well as a good source of protein, pantothenic acid, potassium, iron, zinc, vitamin B6, niacin, phosphorus, and vitamin B1." (*32) One of the most beneficial benefits of consuming sea vegetables regularly is from the high concentrations of iodine found in most varieties. Iodine is a crucial element the body needs to detoxify and sea vegetables contain the highest concentrations of iodine in a bio-available form than found anywhere else on the planet in natural form.

Sea vegetables are great when added to recipes, eaten as a snack, or added to smoothies and juices. Most sea vegetables can be purchased dehydrated or freeze-dried. Look for products with no other ingredients or additives for best results.

Mushrooms

Mushrooms are technically classified as fungus, but often in culinary categories we include them with vegetables so they warrant mentioning here, particularly due to their many health benefits. Of course, we are only referring to mushrooms that are safe for human consumption. Some mushrooms are actually toxic to the body and should be avoided. Those that are considered edible, however, not only taste great and add depth of flavor to any recipe with which they are included, but mushrooms are excellent sources of fiber, selenium, copper, niacin, potassium, phosphorous, B vitamins, vitamin C and iron. "Crimini

AND GOD SAID:

Genesis 27: 37

And Isaac answered Esau, Behold, I have made [Jacob] your lord and master; I have given all his brethren to him for servants, and with corn and [new] wine have I sustained him. (AMV)

Genesis 2: 16

Then the Lord God commanded the man, "You may freely eat fruit from every tree of the orchard."

mushrooms are one of the only natural food sources for vitamin D and one of the few foods that contain germanium." (*33)

Mushrooms have been shown to benefit the body in many ways. For example, mushrooms can boost the immune system, reduce blood pressure, strengthen bones and teeth, lower cholesterol, regulate blood sugar, and reduce the risk of certain cancers like breast cancer and prostrate cancer. Some of our favorite mushrooms include morels, reishi, shitake, cremini, oyster mushrooms, miatake, white button, and portobello.

Some mushrooms, like reishi, miatake, and shitake have additional medicinal benefits such as fighting tumor growth, improving liver function, detoxification, balancing hormones, fighting asthma and allergies, and fighting diabetes. Additionally, reishi mushrooms, in a 2012 study, were shown to support the production of nerve growth factor, a protein that is vital for healthy neurological function and showed promising results in countering the effects of neurodegenerative disorders such as Alzheimer's and Huntington's disease. (*34)

Mushrooms can be eaten raw, however to get the maximum nutritional benefits it is recommended to cook mushrooms before consuming. Mushrooms have cellular walls that are undigestible. By lightly cooking them, this cellular wall is softened and the body is then able to assimilate all that these delicious mushrooms have to offer. Purchase mushrooms when they are fresh (never canned). Store in the refrigerator in a paper bag until ready to use.

How to Prepare and Enjoy Vegetables, Fruits, and Greens

With thousands of varieties of vegetables, fruits, and greens available across the globe we have such a delightful rainbow of colors and flavors from which to choose. Add to that the many ways to prepare them and our plate should never be considered bland or boring. To best enjoy the maximum health benefits these amazing foods have to offer, there are a few methods of preparation that best preserve the nutrient value and "living energy" of the vegetable, fruit, or greens. As a general rule of thumb, some health experts recommend 40-50% of your plate (or more) consisting of vegetables, fruits, or greens. Considering 100% of our diet in the Garden of Eden were these foods, then making them the focal point of the diet makes perfect sense. Here are my top recommendations for preparing vegetables, fruits, and greens:

1. *Raw:* I love eating most fruits, vegetables, and greens raw. Even things like okra and asparagus are amazing right out of the garden. Raw fruits and vegetables, especially when fresh and in-season, have the most nutrients and living energy in them. Not everyone can handle raw, however, especially at first when you are transitioning and healing your digestive system. If this is the case for you, consider starting with the other preparation methods listed, then slowly start adding raw into your diet.

   The mistake I see all too often is thinking a salad every day is the best thing to do when trying to lose weight and get healthy. Don't get me wrong, I love salads and encourage you to enjoy them often... but only if your digestive system can handle them. Unfortunately, many people have been eating processed foods for so long that their digestive bacteria and enzymes are no longer wired to properly handle the workload to break down the fibers of raw foods, especially vegetables. Check with your healthcare provider for recommendations on whether you might benefit from some supplementation like digestive enzymes to assist when consuming raw plant foods. If your digestion can handle it, however, raw is my favorite way to consume most vegetables, fruits, and greens.

   When consuming raw, it is especially important to make sure the fruit or vegetable is at its peak ripeness for best flavor and health benefits. For example, bananas should be eaten when yellow with just a hint of brown spots starting to form. Any green on the skin of the banana indicates that the banana is not ripe and therefore contain more of what are called resistant starches, which are very difficult for most people to digest and can cause pain, bloating, and gas.

   Raw fruits make wonderful desserts and are perfect options when you're craving something sweet. The natural sugars in fruits add intense flavors to any snack or meal. Note: If you are dealing with a candida overgrowth, it is recommended to avoid fruits for a period of time until your candida is no longer a problem. Candida feeds off of sugars, which includes the natural sugars found in all fruits.

   I try to add a little bit of raw into every meal, even if it's just a few sprouts or microgreens, some fresh vegetables, or a small salad. Raw vegetables make wonderful snacks, too. One of my favorite raw snacks is some sprouted hummus with mung spouts and raw cauliflower, bell pepper,

AND GOD SAID:

Exodus 10: 5

...and they shall cover the face of the earth that one will not be able to see the earth, and they shall eat the residue of that which is escaped, which remains unto you from the hail and shall eat every tree which produces fruit for you out of the field:...

AND GOD SAID:

Leviticus 26: 4

Then I will give you rain in due season, and the land shall yield her increase, and the trees of the field shall yield their fruit.

and/or carrots. My daughter's favorite raw snack is snap peas and/or cherry tomatoes. My husband, who is not the most avid vegetable eater, enjoys raw cucumbers, celery, and carrots. There's nothing like a fresh, juicy watermelon on a hot summer day, or the sweet crunch of a fresh apple in the fall. Experiment to find your favorites and if you don't like them the first time, try them again later. Your tastes will change drastically the more you transition to God's way of eating and give your body a chance to rediscover the joy in healthy foods.

2. *Juicing and Smoothies:* Another way to enjoy vegetables, fruits, and greens is by juicing them or making smoothies. This preparation method is an extension of the "raw" category and has literally an infinite number of variations, possibilities, and combinations of recipes. I am a huge fan of juicing and smoothies as they are a delicious way to get your vegetables, fruits, and greens; even for those picky eaters.

The benefits of consuming fresh juices and smoothies are numerous. Juices and smoothies are much easier to digest than their raw counterparts. Juices, especially, are a wonderful way to get an intense dose of nutrients quickly as most of the fiber has been removed during the juicing process. Fiber is an important part of fruits and vegetables, however when making juices and smoothies, we can often consume larger quantities of a larger variety in each cup. Not many of us otherwise could just consume several pounds of vegetables in one sitting. Because juices and smoothies tend to be a mixture of several vegetables and/or fruit, consumers can enjoy foods they wouldn't normally eat or don't like as the flavors of the other ingredients hides the flavors of the individual ingredient. Parents, especially, find benefit from feeding juices and smoothies to their children as a way of getting them to eat more vegetables and greens.

The key to juicing and smoothies is to remember one very important rule of thumb:

Juice your vegetables, blend your fruits, always add greens.

Fruits, even so-called 'sour' fruits, contain much more sugars in the form of fructose than vegetables or greens. Due to their higher level of fruit sugars, it is important to preserve the fiber in the fruits so they don't go

73

through the digestive system too quickly. Also, the amount of sugar in a glass of juice is much more than you would get from eating the fruit; for example we wouldn't normally consume 5 oranges in one sitting... but we would easily drink a cup or two of orange juice. Juicing fruits can lead to quick spikes of blood sugar, insulin issues, and weight gain.

Commercial fruit juices are never recommended, particularly due to the high levels of sugar, the fact that they are no longer "fresh" and the "light energy" is gone from them, and they often contain other harmful ingredients, been pasteurized or processed, or come from concentrate. (More on this in our chapter on sweets.)

Instead of juicing them, fruits can be added to smoothies because they are blended and the fibers of the fruit are included in the final product. Adding a few fruits to a smoothie with lots of greens and some protein makes consuming the final recipe more delicious and enjoyable. A good guideline to remember, is never add more fruits to the smoothie than you would otherwise eat during a single sitting. Again, commercial smoothies are not recommended. There are a few products out there that are in powder form, that were made from carefully preserved ingredients. It is highly recommended to be a smart consumer, researching the ingredients, how they were grown, how they were preserved, how much fruit sugar you are getting in the final product, and how much nutrient value that product is offering.

Vegetables, on the other hand, are wonderful in juices. Combining vegetables and greens in a juice is a great way to quickly and easily get more vegetables into your diet each day. Where it may not be good to get too much fruit at one time due to the sugar content, consuming larger amounts of vegetables and greens can actually be beneficial. As with anything, finding a balance is the key and experimenting to find recipes you and your family enjoys is worth it.

Experts generally all agree that adding more greens to your diet is especially beneficial, particularly dark leafy greens. Adding greens to juices and smoothies add a depth of flavor without being overpowering yet still contribute their "life energy." Excellent greens to add to your juices and smoothies includes kale, spinach, microgreens, sunflower greens, beet greens, turnip greens, chard, collards, parsley, cilantro, wheatgrass, barley grass, purslane, dandelion greens, and sea vegetables (seaweed).

AND GOD SAID:

Joshua 5: 11

On the day after the Passover, on that very day, they ate some of the produce of the land,... (NIV)

Genesis 25: 29

Jacob was cooking vegetable and lentil stew, Esau came in from the field, and he was famished. (NIV)

3. *Lightly Cooked:* The most common way to eat most vegetables (and some fruits and greens) is by lightly cooking them. Cooking softens the cellulose fiber in the food, making them much easier on the digestive process. Lightly cooking changes the flavor profile of foods, making them taste different than their raw counterpart, and in some cases making them more palatable.

Some raw-only advocates will say that cooking destroys important vitamins and minerals, and in some cases that may be partially true, however studies show that only foods that are over-cooked have sufficient nutrient loss to be a concern. In reality, the minor loss of some vitamins and minerals are out-shadowed by the fact that most consumers actually absorb *more* nutrients from lightly cooked foods than raw due to the increase in *bio-available* nutrients and the body's ability to assimilate those nutrients. Maximizing the nutrients and "life energy" found in the foods requires a few considerations when preparing them:

- *How much heat you use.* Heat has been proven to affect nutrients, but unfortunately some heat is required to cook. To maximize nutritional profile, use the lowest heat possible to accomplish the cooking style you are using.
- *How long you cook them.* Going along with the above concept that heat destroys nutrients, even at lower temperatures the nutrients will degrade the longer the cooking time. Keep things as short and sweet as possible.
- *How much water you use.* Certain vitamins and minerals are water-soluble, meaning the nutrients will be leached into the water as it cooks. Cooking in water such as boiling or steaming will naturally lose more water-soluble nutrients than other cooking methods. This is why the water turns green when you steam broccoli, for example.
- *What cooking method you use.* There are many popular techniques for cooking your vegetables, fruits, and greens including steaming, sautéing, baking, roasting, broiling, dehydrating, pressure cooking, and microwaving.

Microwaving has been proven to change the molecular structure of the food cooked, killing all "life energy" found in the food. It is highly recommended to avoid using a microwave for any cooking. Several studies have been conducted where water was microwaved and used to water houseplants. In all cases, the plants watered with microwaved water died. Other studies have shown similar or same results. Consuming any food cooked in a microwave is completely "dead food."

New pressure cooking technology has made old technology of pressure cooking even better and user-friendly. Even those who don't like to cook can quickly, easily, and economically produce delicious results. I'm referring to the Power Pressure Cookers now available. Personally, I think these amazing inventions are the best thing since the advent of the toaster or bread machine! And, best of all, in most cases cooking with a Power Pressure Cooker retains more nutrients than any other cooking method (up to 98%)! If finding the time to cook is one of your biggest stumbling blocks to eating healthy, then you might want to consider trying a Power Pressure Cooker. I can pull frozen chicken out, add some water or broth and a few vegetables and herbs, set the cooker, walk away, and have a delicious and nutritious meal in less than 35 minutes!

Baking, roasting, and broiling offer a unique flavor profile that is truly amazing. If you haven't tried oven-roasting broccoli, brussels sprouts, or cauliflower, I recommend you give it a try. For your convenience I have included the recipe and cooking instructions in our Recipe section. Try this same recipe with sweet potatoes, turnips, carrots, and other root vegetables, too!

Some vegetables like potatoes, sweet potatoes, yams, turnips, rutabaga, and eggplant are best when lightly cooked. The most important thing to remember when cooking your vegetables, fruits, or greens is to enjoy them, regardless of the method used.

4. *Lacto-fermentation:* Another method of preparation for vegetables, fruits, and greens is lacto-fermentation, also sometimes referred to as "culturing". It's unfortunate that lacto-fermentation isn't more commonly known in modern cultures since it was the predominant method of food preservation for thousands of years, preserving the food with natural good bacteria. Cultured foods are probiotic-rich living foods with excellent "life energy" in an easily digestible form. Most commonly recognized versions of lacto-fermented foods include sauerkraut (not the canned version made with vinegar), kimchi, and miso.

AND GOD SAID:

Proverbs 30: 25

The ants are not a strong people, but they prepare their food in the summer.

Isaiah 38: 16

Lord, your discipline is good, for it leads to life and health. You restore my health and allow me to live!

Just about any vegetable, fruit, or green can be lacto-fermented to make delicious snacks, side-dishes, toppings, and condiments. Some of my family's favorite cultured foods include sauerkraut, cultured pickles, cultured radishes, cultured carrots, cultured beets, and cultured garlic. The flavors of lacto-fermented foods tend to be reminiscent of "pickling" without the vinegar or processing and retains most of the bio-available nutrients in the foods; in fact, in many cases the nutrient density is higher than the raw counterpart because the good bacteria work at not only preserving the food, but also "pre-digesting"; meaning they break down the cellular structures making these foods much easier on our digestive system to assimilate.

It is only just recently that medicine and science are starting to fully understand the implications of having a strong, balanced, bacterial flora in the digestive system. Our bodies rely on the good bacteria in our system to perform some pretty key functions that affect our overall sense of health and well-being. Science has linked the good bacteria in our bodies to our immune system, hormones, emotions, and even brain function. Use of antibiotics, use of chemical hand sanitizers and antibacterial soaps, consuming processed foods, taking birth control and certain other medications can all jeopardize the health of the gut flora. One of the best ways to support your good bacteria is to consume lacto-fermented foods because these foods contain numerous strains of good bacteria that helps repopulate the bacteria in your gut. But the best part, is that these foods taste amazing!

The first time I was introduced to lacto-fermented vegetables was at a live workshop led by a leading cultured food expert, Donna Schwenk. During this seminar we got to taste some fabulous examples and hear amazing testimonials of how adding cultured foods helped thousands of people with their health. The most memorable testimonial came from Donna Schwenk herself when she shared how drinking just the *juice* from lacto-fermented sauerkraut helped her with food poisoning within just minutes! That seemed too good to be true. But for the past several years since then, any time anyone in my family starts to get even the slightest stomach upset, we're grabbing a shot glass of sauerkraut juice. And believe it or not, it really does work! Even my husband, who is the biggest skeptic when it comes to natural remedies, will now get his own glass of sauerkraut juice when his stomach is starting to feel off. Whether it's food poisoning, flu, stomach bug, or indigestion... sauerkraut, or rather any lacto-fermented foods or juices, does the trick.

Lacto-fermented foods are super easy and economical to make yourself and don't require any special equipment or fancy ingredients. We have put together an online tutorial that explains all the simple steps in an easy format should you want to learn more and try it yourself. I know you'll love it and be amazed at how easy it is, how delicious the flavors, and how good these foods make you feel! More information on our online course can be found in the Resources section.

If you don't want to make your own, there are many excellent commercial varieties of cultured foods on the market. Look for brands that specify "lacto-fermented" or "living cultures". Most options will be found in the refrigerated section of your grocery store and should only contain a few ingredients like water and sea salt.

Regardless of how you prepare them, whether raw, in smoothies or juices, lightly cooked, or lacto-fermented, you'll want to return to the Garden of Eden and enjoy vegetables, fruits, and greens as much as possible. The more colorful a variety you consume, the more diverse nutrients and phytonutrients, with their "life energy", that you will assimilate. As a result, you body will have the tools it needs to repair and heal, detoxify, regenerate and thrive.

Current food pyramid guidelines say we should be consuming a minimum of 5-7 servings per day of vegetables, fruits, and greens. Keep in mind that this is the minimum recommendations. It is very difficult to "over-eat" these foods with all their amazing benefits and "life energy!"

But I (...my spouse...my kids...) don't like vegetables!

About now, some of you may be thinking, "yeah, that's great and all, but I don't like vegetables." Or, you may be saying, "my kid's are picky eaters and won't eat vegetables." If this is you, take heart and read on. There is definitely hope for you!

Often, when someone tells me they don't like vegetables, my next question is which vegetables have you tried, where did you get them, and how were they prepared? Generally I'll get responses like salad, canned peas, canned asparagus, carrots, or broccoli. Ok, I get it. But honestly if *my* only experience with vegetables was canned peas or what is served at the schools, then I would say I don't like vegetables either.

AND GOD SAID:

Matthew 12: 33

Either make the tree good and its fruit good, or make the tree bad and its fruit bad; for the tree is known by its fruit.

Genesis 28: 3

And may God, the Ruler of all, give you his blessing, giving you fruit and increase, so that you may become an army of peoples.

My husband says he doesn't like tomatoes. In truth, he eats tomatoes all the time. There are over 15,000 documented varieties of tomatoes grown worldwide in colors ranging from the traditional red to yellow, orange, green, white, black, blue, striped, and speckled in sizes from tiny cherry tomatoes to several pound whoppers. Each variety has a much different flavor profile. Add to that how much the flavor of a tomato changes when it is juiced, cooked, lacto-fermented, or added to sauces and you have an almost infinite number of tastes and ways you can enjoy them. And, the majority of the flavor from a vegetable or fruit comes from the minerals found in them. A tomato from the store, grown in commercial fields or greenhouses, picked when they are green to transport them, and then gassed to turn them red will never have the flavor of a vine-ripened tomato, grown in rich, organic soil, and picked at the peak of freshness.

Peas are another excellent example. Raw peas have a completely different taste than canned peas, steamed peas, sautéed peas, or pea sprouts. If you don't think you like peas, have you tried them in other methods or varieties?

And, with literally hundreds of thousands of types of vegetables, fruits, and greens on this planet coupled with the even greater number should you break that down into unique varieties, plus the methods of preparation for each type of vegetable, fruit, or green, and you have so many flavor options that you are bound to find at least *some* that you like. You just have to do a little experimenting and be willing to keep trying until you find your favorites. And, you will find that the more you transition away from the sugar-laden goodies or processed foods, your taste preferences will change and you may even find yourself CRAVING those vegetables!

In the meantime, you can still "sneak" a few additional varieties into juices or smoothies that they won't even know are there! Cooked cauliflower or sweet potatoes can be added to casseroles or pasta dishes and they won't even taste them. Kale, spinach, microgreens, and other greens can be easily added to soups, smoothies, and casseroles. Be creative and keep trying.

For kids, including them in the shopping, meal prep, and if possible growing of vegetables, fruits, and greens will encourage them even more. Participation, for some reason, adds to their willingness to eat things they otherwise normally wouldn't. I was talking with a good friend of mine recently, who happens to be my next door neighbor. She said she has so much trouble getting her son to eat healthy because he's such a "picky eater." Honestly, I was surprised when she told me this, because all summer whenever he would come over to our house and play outside with the neighborhood kids, I would see them in the garden happily munching on whatever was ripe for picking. Kids especially seem to be naturally drawn to watching things grow...and when they do, it is rare to see a child not find enjoyment from eating the "fruits" of their labor. (Pun intended.)

Even if you don't have space for a garden, there are many options available where you can grow *some* things. Sprouts, microgreens, and herbs can be grown right in your kitchen. Tomatoes, peppers, cucumbers, potatoes, strawberries and many others can be grown in pots on a porch or deck. New technology like tower gardens that use hydroponics or aeroponics work well for expanding your growing options year round, indoors. There's nothing like the expressions on the faces of the kiddos when they participate in growing and then eat things like strawberries, tomatoes, and cucumbers right off the plant.

But I can't afford to eat lots of vegetables, fruits, and greens...

Hey, I get it. You may be thinking that eating lots of vegetables, fruits, and greens is out of your budget. If this is you, take heart. I'm going to share with you some ways you can still stay within budget while eating healthy!

1. *Reallocation of funds:* First, you may be surprised at how much money you *save* by eating healthy! When you stop buying all those pre-package processed foods, chemically-laden toxic soft drinks, and other "dead foods", you free up tons of cash to use for better choices.
2. *Grow what you can:* Planting a garden is a wonderful way to get fresh produce without much money out of pocket. Seeds are extremely economical and with just a little bit of effort will yield a bounty of food for your table. Surplus can be preserved for later enjoyment to save even more throughout the year.
3. *Buy in bulk when possible:* Generally, when fruits and vegetables are in season, you can purchase them much more economically at farmers markets, grocers, and co-ops. If you can, buy extra and freeze or preserve it for later use.
4. *Shop local farmers markets:* Most communities have farmers markets where you can buy local, fresh produce. Generally, since you are buying direct from the grower, you can cut out the middle-man and get much better prices.
5. *Shop Online:* Some things can be found more economically online.

AND GOD SAID:

Deuteronomy 6: 24

The Lord commanded us to follow all these statutes and to fear the Lord our God for our prosperity always and for our preservation.

John 15: 4-5

Abide in Me and I in you. As the branch cannot bear fruit of itself unless it abides in the vine, so neither can you unless you abide in Me. (ASV)

6. *Shop Bulk/Discount stores:* When buying frozen produce especially, I find I can get some really great prices when I shop the bigger discount stores.

A Word About "Organic"

Part of eating healthy according to God's Plan is to reduce the amount of toxic exposure your body must deal with in the food you are eating. At one time, the simple solution was to just choose "organic" when purchasing vegetables, fruits, and greens. Where this is in most cases generally true, it is not *always* worth the extra money you are paying for organic. Let me explain.

"Organic" simply means that the vegetable or fruit was grown and processed using natural substances and methods. Farms that grow and label their product as "organic" must go through rigorous organic certification processes including on-site inspections of seed sources, soil conditions, crop health, weed and pest management, water systems, contamination risks, and record-keeping. (*35) The process of getting USDA Organic Certified is expensive and time-consuming, partly accounting for the higher prices of organic goods.

Organic produce grown outside the United States and imported, however, may have been *grown* organically without the use of harmful pesticides; but current U.S. Regulation requires all produce brought across our borders to be sprayed to avoid bringing in any harmful pathogens from another country. Therefore, your bell peppers from Mexico that were grown organically and that you paid almost twice the price for, still have toxic pesticides and chemicals that need to be carefully removed prior to consuming. Watch your labels and where the produce was grown.

On labels, if a product says "made with organic", regulations state that at least 70% of the final product have to have been organically produced. The remaining ingredients do not have to follow the organic standards.

The regulations for organic are beneficial and help us as consumers have a better idea of where our food is coming from and how it was grown. There's no substitute for growing your own or buying from local farmers where you can talk to them about their growing practices, ask them questions, and in some cases even visit their farms. Many local farms don't go through the trouble of getting organic certified even though they use organic practices. So choose organic when you can, yet being mindful of where it was grown, how it was handled, and how far it had to travel to get to your table.

What about lectins found in vegetables and grains? Are they really harmful?

Recently, there has been quite a bit of advertising about lectins in foods, particularly vegetables in the nightshade family like tomatoes, peppers, eggplant, and potatoes, as well as beans, grains, dairy, certain seafood, peanuts, and cashews. Is this true? Well, yes and no. The answer is not exactly black and white, which makes the question of lectins a controversial one. Science is just now starting to do more research surrounding lectins, and hopefully over time we will have a clearer understanding. Based on the research I have seen, here is my interpretation of what you need to know.

Lectins are a type of protein that can bind to cell membranes and offer a way for molecules to stick together without getting the immune system involved. In some cases, this can actually be beneficial to the body, but when consumed in excess, can disrupt the digestive system and contribute to inflammation. Lectins are found primarily in seeds, grains, beans, nuts, and legumes and are believed to be part of a plant's natural defense system against insects, pests, and microorganisms. Lectins also help the seed remain intact as it passes through an animals' digestive system.

Scientists have found lectins to be resistant to human digestion and they can enter the bloodstream unchanged. Because we don't digest lectins well, some people may produce antibodies to them, creating an immune response. Scientists have further found that certain seeds, like kidney beans, contain higher amounts of lectins, so much so that consuming even as few as four raw kidney beans can trigger a massive digestive response. Seeds that have been genetically modified, like GMO wheat and corn also contain considerably higher amounts of lectins.

These recent studies on lectins just lend more weight to what we have already discussed in the importance of sprouting or soaking grains, seeds, nuts, and legumes before consuming them, as this process greatly reduces, or completely neutralizes the harmful effects of lectins. But what about the nightshades like tomatoes and peppers?

First, it is important to listen to your body. If you find yourself reacting to these foods then by all means consider cutting them from your diet. Also, choose

AND GOD SAID.

Psalm 136: 25

He gives food to every creature. His love endures forever.

Galatians 5: 22-23

But the fruit of the Spirit is love, joy, peace, forbearance, kindness, goodness, faithfulness, gentleness, and self-control. (NIV)

heirloom varieties that have not been genetically changed or hybridized. If lectins are a concern or if you are suffering from digestive issues or chronic weight issues, you might also consider removing the skins and seeds, and cooking them thoroughly rather than eating them raw until your digestive system has a chance to re-balance. Then you can try slowly reintroducing these foods, listening carefully to your body. Ultimately, it is your body, and through prayer, God will guide you on what is best for you.

The Spiritual Significance of Fruit

Although this chapter delves into the importance physically of vegetables, fruits, and greens, spiritually our emphasis for discussion here will be specifically on fruit alone. Fruit has deep spiritual meaning in the Bible and is mentioned hundreds of times, particularly in cases of spiritual significance.

Why does God not use vegetables for spiritual metaphors as much as fruits? Personally, I can't help but feel that God uses fruits to emphasize his points over vegetables for several reasons. Even though vegetables physically are proven to be the foundation for health, fruits are so much sweeter and have a much more positive feel for most of us. Face it. We know we should eat our vegetables, but we rarely crave a carrot or a radish like we do blueberries or a sweet, juicy orange. We are more drawn to the sweetness and enjoyment of fruits, just as we are naturally drawn to a deeper connection with God.

Also...and more importantly, fruits by definition are generally a sweet pulp or plant substance that protects the seed until new life can be brought forth. Vegetables, on the other hand, tend to be parts of the plant (roots, stalks, pods, tubers, leaves, etc.) The fruit is what brings forth a hope for the future and the new life that springs forth from its seeds. This fundamental hope for new life and a desire for a better future deeply correlates with the messages in both the Old Testament and the New Testament including the promises of eternal life through Jesus Christ.

In Matthew 7: 20, Jesus says, "You will recognize them by their fruits." When we draw near to Him and develop a deep relationship with Christ, we produce good "fruits" that are sweet, wholesome, and nourishing; meaning we personify (as best we can, as we are all flawed and fall short) the message of Jesus. The bible often uses the representation or metaphor of fruit to describe the produce of our lives. What we produce can either be good or it can be bad, depending on our direction and our priorities.

"Fruit is the direct result of whatever controls our hearts. (Matthew 15:19). The fruit of a life not surrendered to Jesus includes 'sexual immortality, impurity and debouchery, idolatry and wichcraft, hatred, discord, jealousy, fits of rage,' and many other evil acts (Galatians 5: 19-20). In contrast, the fruit of the Spirit of God is 'love, joy, peace, patience, kindness, goodness, faithfulness, gentleness, and self-control' (Galatians 5: 22-23)." (*36)

We must seek to produce good fruits by drawing closer to God, as it is through our relationship with Him that we can keep our priorities right and our hearts pure. A life centered on self will not produce good fruits. It is only when we turn outwards and serve others can we fully appreciate and experience the true depth of love, joy, peace, patience, kindness, goodness, gentleness, and self-control.

Once we have mastered our self-control and begun to draw closer to God, he calls us to have a higher purpose than ourselves. In John 15: 16, Jesus says, "You did not choose me, but I chose you and appointed you to go and bear fruit; fruit that will last." In this verse, bearing fruit that will last means we are to share what we know so that others too may draw closer to God, thus they too may find the true joy and peace that comes from Him. The fruit you produce becomes your legacy; will your legacy be good fruit or bad fruit?

AND GOD SAID:

Galatians 5: 22-23

But the fruit of the Spirit is love, joy, peace, patience, kindness, goodness, faithfulness, gentleness, and self-control.

Theologenic Diet
Vegetables, Fruits, and Greens

The following is a summary of foods you can enjoy as discussed in this chapter. This list is by no means complete as there are thousands of varieties available, yet is meant as a basic guideline to get you started and show you the diversity of healthy options available.

Vegetables:
Acorn Squash
Artichoke
Asparagus (Green and Purple)
Avocado
Bamboo Shoots
Beans
Beets (Red, White, Orange, Yellow)
Belgian Endive
Bitter Melon
Bok Choy
Broadbeans (Fava Beans)
Broccoli
Brussel Sprouts
Butternut Squash
Cabbage (Green, & Red/Purple)
Carrots (Yellow, White, Red, & Orange)
Cassava (Yuca Root)
Cauliflower (White, Purple, Orange)
Celeriac (Celery Root)
Celery
Corn
Crookneck Squash
Cucumber
Daikon Radish
Edamame
Eggplant
Endive
Fennel
Garlic
Ginger Root
Horseradish
Jalapeno
Jerusalem Artichoke
Jicama
Kohlrabi
Leeks
Okra (Green, Purple)
Onions (White, Yellow, Red)
Parsnip
Peas

Pepper, Sweet (Red, Orange, Yellow, Green, Purple, Brown)
Pepper, Hot
Potato (White, Yellow, Red)
Pumpkin
Radiccio
Radish (Red, White, Pink, Yellow, Orange)
Rutabaga
Salsify
Shallots
Snow Peas
Spaghetti Squash
Sweet Potato (Orange, Purple)
Tomatillo (Green, Purple)
Tomato (Red, Orange, Yellow, Green, Purple, Black, Striped, Speckled)
Turnip
Water Chestnuts
Yam
Zucchini

Greens:
Arugula
Beet Greens
Broccoli Rabe
Chicory (Curly Endive)
Collards
Dandelion Greens
Kale
Lettuce
Mustard Greens
Purslane
Spinach
Sorrel
Stinging Nettle
Sweet Potato Greens
Swish Chard
Watercress

Microgreens:
Alfalfa
Basil Greens
Beet Greens
Broccoli
Celery
Chard
Chia
Cilantro
Clover
Dill
Flax
Kale
Kohlrabi
Lettuce
Mustard Greens
Pea Shoots
Sunflower Greens
Turnip Greens

Mushrooms:
Chanterelle
Chicken of the Woods
Cremini
Maitake
Morels
Oyster
Portobello
Reishi
Shitake
Truffles
White Button

Sea Vegetables (Seaweed)
Nori
Kelp
Dulse
Wakame
Kombu
Agar agar
Hijiki

Fruits:
Apple
Apricot
Acai
Acerola
Banana

Bayberry
Blueberry
Blackberry
Boysenberry
Bearberry
Bilberry
Black Cherry
Black Raspberry
Cantaloupe
Cherry
Chokeberry
Coconut
Cranberry
Currant
Date
Dragon Fruit
Elderberry
Fig
Goji Berry
Gooseberry
Grapes
Grapefruit
Guava
Hackberry
Hawthorn
Honeydew
Honeysuckle
Huckleberry
Jackfruit
Juniper Berry
Kiwi
Humquat
Lemon
Lime
Lingonberry
Loganberry
Lychee
Mandarin
Mangosteen
Nectarine
Olive
Oranges
Papaya
Passion Fruit
Peach
Pear
Persimmon
Pineapple

...Fruits (continued)

Pineberry
Plum
Pluot
Pomegranate
Pomelo
Raspberry
Star Fruit

Strawberry
Tamarind
Tangelo
Ugli
Vanilla
Watermelon

Chapter Summary:

The cornerstone to a healthy, biblically-based diet are the foods given to us from the beginning of time in the Garden of Eden. This includes vegetables, fruits, and greens. The reason these foods are so healthy and why they support health more than any other category of food is the amount of "life energy" found in them. Only plant-based foods contain phytonutrients which are the foundation to maintaining optimum health. Best of all, these foods are delicious, economical, and easy to prepare. To maximize the diversity of phytonutrient benefits, regularly consume more colors through a variety of vegetables, fruits,and greens.

Action Items:

1. Be aware of how much "life energy" foods you are consuming and start increasing the variety and quantity of vegetables, fruits, and greens you are enjoying each day. Make it your goal that at least 40% or more of the plate contains these foods.
2. Add more color to your plate. See how many colors you can get into your diet through vegetables, fruits, and greens. Try new kinds and explore new varieties to 'eat the rainbow' every day. Ever try a purple carrot or yellow watermelon?
3. Start planning your weekly menus (We have conveniently included a few suggested menu plans in this book to help you get started). Planning ahead means you will have the groceries on hand for healthy meals, save time, reduce to tendency to just grab unhealthy "convenience" foods, and stay committed to this new way of approaching your food.
4. Make a point to share "good fruits" each day with someone through kindness, thoughtfulness, generosity, love, forgiveness, or any of the other fruits of the Spirit. When you find yourself getting "rotten" and bearing "bad fruits", turn to God for guidance and forgiveness, then move forward with "good fruit."

AND GOD SAID:

John 15: 16

You did not choose me, but I chose you and appointed you to go and bear fruit; fruit that will last. (NIV)

Notes:

Chapter 7: God's Word on Meat

Physical Significance of Meat

To meat or not to meat, that is the question. The subject of eating meat is sometimes quite controversial and one that I often get questions about. If you are currently a vegan (eat no animal products) or vegetarian (don't eat meat), then by all means continue (as long as you are consuming a well-balanced diet and getting enough protein through legumes and other sources.

If you do currently eat meat, you'll want to read this chapter with an open mind as I am going to point out several key considerations about eating meat that God is VERY clear about. My goal is not to convince you one way or the other, but rather to educate you about God's very specific guidelines on eating meat and the science behind why these laws and guidelines are so important for us to follow, even in our modern world. I get more resistance and arguments about this topic than any other presented in this book, as people become quite passionate about their choices, one way or the other. Regardless of your position, just consider getting the facts with an open mind, and then turn to God for answers on what is best for you.

Meat can be quite nutritious and benefit the body through the amino acids (building blocks) found in the protein. However, more than with any other food choice, meat has changed drastically since Biblical times in the genetics, the cultural practices, and the preparation of the meat dishes, leading to detrimental mistakes that harm the body, opening a pathway for disease. The most common mistakes I see when eating meat; mistakes that turn what would otherwise be a healthy addition to your diet into something potentially toxic or unhealthy, often include:
- Choosing the wrong kinds of meats.
- Eating too much meat in a meal.
- Eating meat that has been grown in "unhealthy" conditions or unhealthy processing practices.
- Eating processed meats that have chemical additives or other unhealthy ingredients added.

Let's take a look at each of these common mistakes, along with God's words and what science says about meat, so you can make better decisions that will support your health.

AND GOD SAID:

Isaiah 25: 6

On this mountain the Lord Almighty will prepare a feast of rish food for all peoples, a banquet of aged wine- the best of meats and the finest of wines. (NIV)

Genesis 7: 1 - 3

The Lord then said to Noah, "Go into the ark, you and your whole family, because I have found you righteous in this generation. Take with you seven pairs of every kind of clean animal, a male and its mate, and one pair of every kind of unclean animal, a male and its mate, and also seven pairs of every kind of bird, to keep their various kinds alive throughout the earth.

Mistake #1: Choosing the wrong kinds of meats.

As we mentioned in the previous chapter, in the beginning when we were in the Garden of Eden we only ate fruits, vegetables, herbs, nuts, and greens. For thousands of years, man lived primarily as vegetarians and had healthy lives, often living for hundreds of years! Methuselah lived to the ripe old age of 969! It wasn't until the Flood when Noah and his family entered the ark with all the animals that meat as a food is mentioned in the Bible. Why did meat suddenly become a part of our diets when for so long man lived well off just vegetative foods?

Some biblical scholars believe that for one, man had no choice. When the earth was covered with water, sea life thrived but all vegetation on the planet perished along with the animals and people not on the ark. God gave us a viable alternative that Noah and his family could use as food to sustain them during the years until they could once again enjoy fresh vegetation. Although the Bible isn't specific, surely Noah and his family included rations of grains, seeds, nuts, and some preserved fruits and vegetables, however they would have been limited on what they could store, especially for such a long voyage.

Once the waters started to recede, it would take years before plant life would fully recover. As a homesteader I am deeply aware of the time it takes to plant something, watch it grow, and wait for it to produce, which can take incredible patience and perseverance. Especially in the case of trees, it can even take decades before that tree will start to produce food for us to eat. For example, a pecan tree from seed to edible nut can take about 20 years or more!

No one knows for sure why the life-span of man went from living hundreds of years prior to the Flood to about 120 years after the Flood, but some scholars have speculated. A few theologians believe that during pre-fall times the nutrient density of the soil and vegetation were much more concentrated. The Flood diluted these nutrients, spreading them across the globe.

Iodine is one example of this intense dilution. Iodine is absorbed and used in many areas of the body, with deficiencies causing a multitude of health issues. Some key areas of the body that use large amounts of iodine include the thyroid, women's ovaries, bone marrow, breasts, salivary glands, pancreas, muscles, stomach, cerebral spinal fluid, the skin, and the brain. A deficiency of iodine is not uncommon, especially in areas further inland that don't regularly consume ocean foods. Ever since the Flood, our primary iodine sources come from the sea in the form of fish and seaweeds.

Other scholars will argue that the life-span reduced so drastically because man started eating meat. There is no scientific evidence to prove this, however, and the reality is that the body needs protein in order to survive and thrive. Where it is true that it is possible to get all 20 essential amino acids of protein from vegetative sources, they do not contain all 20 which requires much more creativity and care on meal planning for vegetarians and vegans to ensure these nutritional needs are met. Meat, on the other hand, does contain all 20 essential amino acids. Essential amino acids are those that the body is unable to produce itself, rather requiring consumption of foods containing them to meet this need. Meat also contains important other nutrients like iron, zinc, and selenium.

I had a doctor tell me one time that it is important to include meat in the diet. His approach was that the nutritional benefits of meat help with key body functions such as healing and repair. The 20 essential amino acids found in meats make up the building blocks for regeneration. His clinical studies showed better recovery with meat-eating patients over vegan patients.

The key to eating meats, however is choosing meats that have been approved by God. In choosing which meats to consume, God was *very specific* about which animals were "clean" and which were "unclean". Starting in Leviticus 11: 2, the instructions given to Moses and Aaron by God were:

> *...of all animals that live on land, these are the ones you may eat: you may eat any animal that has a divided hoof and that chews the cud. There are some that only chew the cud or only have a divided hoof, but you must not eat them. The camel, though it chews the cud does not have a divided hoof; it is ceremonially unclean for you. The rabbit, though it chews the cud, does not have a divided hoof; it is unclean for you. And the pig, though it has a divided hoof, does not chew the cud; it is unclean for you. You must not eat their meat or touch their carcasses; they are unclean for you.*

> *Of all the creatures living in the water of the seas and the streams you may eat any that have fins and scales. But all creatures in the seas or streams that do not have fins and scales- whether among all the swarming things or among all the other living creatures in the water- you*

AND GOD SAID:

Leviticus 11: 2

...of all animals that live on land, these are the ones you may eat:... (NIV)

Leviticus 11: 46- 47

You must distinguish between the unclean and the clean, between living creatures that may be eaten and those that may not be eaten. (NIV)

are to regard as unclean. And since you are to regard them as unclean, you must not eat their meat; you must regard their carcasses as unclean. Anything living in the water that does not have fins and scales is to be regarded as unclean by you.

These are the birds you are to regard as unclean and not eat because they are unclean: the eagle, the vulture, the red kite, any kind of black kite, any kind of raven, the owl, the osprey, the stork, any kind of heron, the hoopoe and the bat.

All flying insects that walk on all fours are to be regarded as unclean by you. There are, however, some flying insects that walk on all fours that you may eat: those that have jointed legs for hopping on the ground. Of these you may eat any kind of locust, katydid, cricket, or grasshopper. But all other flying insects that have four legs you are to regard as unclean...

...Of the animals that move along the ground, these are unclean to you: the weasel, the rat, any kind of lizard. Of all those that move along the ground, these are unclean for you...

These are the regulations concerning animals, birds, every living thing that moves about in the water and every creature that moves along the ground. You must distinguish between the unclean and the clean, between living creatures that may be eaten and those that may not be eaten." (Leviticus 11: 2-47 NIV)

These verses in Leviticus are one of many areas in scripture that offer specific guidelines about our diet. What is so interesting to me, is that God is more specific about meat than any other food category. He goes into great detail so that there can be no misunderstanding or confusion. These words are quite clear on which meats are good for us and which ones are not. What I also find interesting is that if you look at the teachings of other primary religions, each has almost identical guidelines regarding "clean" and "unclean" meats. For your convenience, I have included a very clear list at the end of this chapter to help you differentiate between what is mentioned is these verses as "clean" meats according to what you find in the grocery stores today.

"Clean" meats include red meats such as beef, veal, venison, lamb, mutton, and chevron, white meats such as chicken, turkey, and quail, and seafood choices from fish with scales and fins like cod, tuna, and salmon.

With so many choices offered to us in the "clean" categories, we should have no trouble following God's plan and still have a diverse diet. Unfortunately, however, several categories of "unclean" meats are also some of the most common to grace the modern table. These off-limits meats include all pork including ham, bacon, sausage, pork ribs, pork chops, pork roast, pepperoni, hot dogs made with pork, and any other pork-based products, and all shellfish including shrimp, crab, scallops, oysters, and lobster.

Having been raised on a regular fare of these foods, I was resistant at first to "give up" what I had come to perceive as "pantry items." Why would God say, "No," to so many foods that we have come to love and consume regularly? To understand the answer to this question, we again turn to science.

When differentiating between "clean" and "unclean" meats, it is interesting to note that the clean meats generally eat grasses, plants, and grains; offering one layer of separation from the original "life-energy" captured by the sun into plant tissues. In contrast, "almost all of the creatures on the unclean list are scavengers. In many cases they don't hunt for their own food; they eat the dead and decaying matter of our environment. A catfish does that at the bottom of a pond; lobsters and shrimp do it in the ocean. A pig will eat anything. Vultures, almost by definition, are known for their scavenger habits... [Also], an animal doesn't have to be a scavenger to be unclean. Horses and rabbits, for example, are unclean because they do not have split hooves. Although they are considered to be good food in some [cultures], studies have shown that horse meat often contains viruses and parasites. Rabbits, as innocent as they appear, are the cause of tularemia (an infectious disease) in humans.... Shrimp, oysters, crab, scallops, and mussels are particularly efficient at [purifying their environment].... Chemicals, toxins, harmful bacteria, parasites, and viruses become concentrated in [their tissues] " (*39).

When God gave permission for us to eat meat, the red meats He specifies as allowed are those coming from animals who both chew the cud and have cloven hooves. Animals that "chew the cud" are herbivores (meaning they only eat plant-based foods like grasses and some grains) and they have multiple stomachs with which to better digest the plant fibers. These animals are often referred to as "ruminants." Because ruminants have multiple stomachs, they tend to have a

AND GOD SAID:

Romans 14: 6

Whoever regards one day as special does so to the Lord. Whoever eats meat does so to the Lord, for they give thanks to God; and whoever abstains does so to the Lord and gives thans to God. (NIV)

Mark 7: 17-19

... Nothing that enters a person from the outside can defile them. For it doesn't go into their heart but into their stomach, and then out of the body. (NIV)

much more efficient digestive system than those animals with single stomachs, which means that they not only are more effective at converting plant energy into usable forms and then storing that energy in their fat and muscle tissues, but they also have a much better filtration system to avoid toxins and parasites from permeating into the fat and muscle tissues.

Pigs, however, may have cloven hooves but they only have one stomach and are considered omnivores (meaning they eat plant-based foods AND animal-based foods). The digestive system of pigs is very similar to ours, in that their single stomach is very acidic. "Pigs are gluttonous, never knowing when to stop eating. Their stomach acids become diluted because of the volume of food, allowing all kinds of vermin to pass through this protective barrier. Parasites, bacteria, viruses, and toxins can pass into the pig's flesh because of overeating. These toxins and infectious agents can be passed on to humans when they eat a pig's flesh" (*37). Currently, in the United States, three of the six most common food-borne parasitic diseases of humans are associated with pork consumption.

In his book, *What Would Jesus Eat*, Dr. Don Colbert adds: "Besides being gluttons, swine are also extremely filthy animals. They will eat garbage, feces, and even decaying flesh. All that is eaten usually becomes part of the pig's own flesh... Aside from the diseases routinely carried by swine, pork is also a very fatty meat. The toxins in pork are held especially in the fat, which is not isolated from the meat as can be the case in lean beef, but rather, it is dispersed throughout the meat" (*38).

A common misconception is to assume that God told us not to eat pork because the technology of the time was inferior to what it is today, and now we have better ways of preparing and cooking the meat to negate these problems. This is not the case, however. Many of the toxins, diseases, and parasites associated with pork consumption are *not* eliminated during the cooking process. Moreover, archaeological discoveries in ancient Israelites' ruins have uncovered some very sophisticated ovens and cooking devices, indicating a clear knowledge of the importance of cooking meat. Cooking methods does not make an unclean meat clean, nor does how that animal was raised. God does not say that pork can be made clean through certain circumstances. Rather he is very clear that pork is unclean and should be avoided.

Another misconception is that the New Testament teachings, particularly as seen in Mark 7: 17-19 when Jesus said "...nothing that enters a person from the outside can defile them. For it doesn't go into their heart but into their stomach, and then out of the body"; negates all laws and rules set forth in the Old Testament. This thinking is flawed, however, when we look deeper into scripture to best interpret what is meant by these verses. The New International Version of the Bible and the New American Standard Bible will end verse 19 with: "(In saying this, Jesus declared all foods 'clean')." This doesn't mean that we can ignore God's clear law on which meats are good for us and which are not, however. Both these versions add this statement in parenthesis "()" indicating they were added by the translator as his/her *interpretation*. Both the King James Version and the New King James Version "indicate that the bodily digestive process purifies food as opposed to Jesus making a pronouncement reversing God's laws on which meats to eat." (*39)

> In fact, "*from cover to cover, from Genesis to Revelation, nowhere in the Bible do we find an example of a servant of God or follower of Jesus Christ eating the flesh of an unclean animal. If at any time the distinctions between clean and unclean meats had ceased to exist, shouldn't that have been made clear in the Bible through the example of God's servants?*

> *On the contrary, well into the time of the early Church we find Christ's followers scrupulously avoiding eating animal flesh that God had revealed as being unclean (Acts 10:14; 11:8). Prophecies of the time of the end make the same distinctions (Revelation 18:2; Isaiah 66: 15-17). (*39)

Still not convinced? Let's take a quick look at a telling event from Jesus' Ministry:

> *Many people assume that Jesus Christ abolished the distinctions between clean and unclean meats, even though, as we have seen, no evidence for this exists in the Scriptures. However, the Bible includes a report of a telling incident that shows whether Jesus viewed pigs as suitable for food.*

> *Before we examine that account, let's understand a part of Christ's character–that He apparently was never wasteful. On two occasions during His ministry, Jesus miraculously multiplied a few fish and loaves of bread to feed large crowds that followed Him; on one occasion 4,000 and the other 5,000 strong (Matthew 14: 15-21; 15: 32-38). But, in spite of an abundance of food, Christ did not allow any of it to go to waste. "So*

AND GOD SAID:

Acts 10: 14

"Surely not, Lord!" Peter replied. "I have never eaten anything impure or unclean."

Hebrews 13: 8

Jesus Christ is the same yesterday and today and forever. (NIV)

when they [the crowds] were filled, He said to His disciples, 'Gather up the fragments that remain, so that nothing is lost'" (John 6:12).

The disciples gathered up 12 baskets of leftover food after the first of these miracles and seven after the second. He specifically told His disciples not to allow any of it to be thrown away.

With the understanding that Jesus was compassionate and not wasteful toward food, let's examine an incident involving Him and some unclean animals– a large herd of pigs.

Mark 5: 1-13 records that Jesus crossed the Sea of Galilee by boat to the region of Gadara, a gentile (non-Jewish) area on the eastern shore. There He was met by a demon-possessed man from whom He would shortly cast many evil spirits.

In this remarkable encounter, the demons requested that Jesus send them into a herd of 2,000 swine on a nearby hillside. Jesus granted their request, and, when the demons entered the swine, "the herd ran violently down the steep place into the sea, and drowned in the sea" (Mark 5: 13).

Many have puzzled over this astounding incident in which Jesus precipitated the destruction of a valuable herd of 2,000 pigs–enough to feed many thousands of people. Yet we should not be surprised when we understand the biblical instruction that these animals should never have been raised for food, and their owner was acting in defiance of God's laws.

Beyond question is that Jesus didn't consider the swine to be suitable for food–even for the gentiles of this area. The compassionate Savior of mankind, the one who ordered scraps of bread and fish to be gathered up so none would go to waste, would never have wasted such a valuable resource had He considered the pigs to be an acceptable part of the human diet.

*Jesus is "the same yesterday, today, and forever" (Hebrews 13:8). Animals He viewed as unfit for human consumption 2,000 years ago remain unfit for us to eat in our day. (*39)*

It is clear that God loves us and wants what is best for us, which is why he gives us these clear guidelines about meat. Unclean meats come from animals that God put on the earth to clean up the toxins, waste, and sludge of the world; or He identified them as unclean because they carry diseases. These animals serve a purpose; just not on the dinner table.

Mistake #2: Eating too much meat in a meal.

God often warns us in scripture about gluttony and the dangers it brings to us both physically and spiritually. Another common mistake when eating meat is the consumption of too much meat at a given time. This mistake becomes increasingly common as our culture has evolved into one of 12 ounce and 16 ounce steaks, super-sized burgers, and double-meat combos.

Granted, meat provides a good source of protein and essential amino acids, the building blocks for bone, cartilage, muscle, skin, hormones, and enzymes, but too much meat during a meal is difficult for the digestive system to handle. I had a renowned nutrition doctor tell me that a good rule of thumb in knowing how much meat your digestive system can efficiently handle is equivalent to the size of the palm of the hand, or around 4-6 ounces per meal. This simple statement he made offered me a much faster and easier visual on how much meat I should have on my plate. Consuming more than that, and the body cannot produce sufficient enzymes and acids to fully break down the meat, often resulting in bloating, nausea, gas, indigestion, heartburn, constipation, or weight gain. Long-term effects may include excessive body odor, IBS (Irritable Bowel Syndrome), heart disease, high blood pressure, high cholesterol, and certain types of cancers.

Some experts will further recommend limiting red meat to only about 2-3 times per month, opting for lighter meat choices such as poultry and fish as better regular choices. In Scripture, red meat was generally reserved for special occasions and feasts; (prepare the fatted calf).

Most of the time, we have it backwards. Many Americans consume red meats almost daily and fish rarely. Although clean red meats are excellent choices nutritionally, fish, particularly oily, cold water fish, contains higher amounts of valuable Omega Fatty Acids, particularly Omega-3. Regular consumption of omega fatty acids, in balance, help with brain function, vision, moods, hormones, and the immune system. So enjoy your clean meats, but keep the portions to the size of your palm and diversify which clean meats you regularly enjoy.

AND GOD SAID:

Exodus 16: 8

Moses also said, "You will know that it was the Lord when he gives you meat to eat in the evening and all the bread you want in the morning, because he has heard your grumbling against him. Who are we? You are not grumbling agains us, but against the Lord."

Ezekiel 24: 10

So heap on the wood and kindle the fire. Cook the meat well, mixing in the spices; and let the bones be charred.

Mistake #3: Eating meat that has been grown in "unhealthy" conditions or unhealthy processing practices.

Unfortunately, it is necessary to take a moment to address where your meat comes from. The most important choices when buying meat are what kind and how much as we already discussed, however, where that meat comes from and how it was raised, processed, and handled *does* play a role in how healthy that meat may be.

As the world gets smaller, populations rise, and consumerism continues to dominate, agriculture has changed to accommodate. Small family farms are rare, being replaced by large corporate farms. Larger farms tend to adopt practices focused on rapid growth to maximize profits. How the animals are housed, what they are fed, medications they receive, and other decisions are a result of years of study in efficiency and profit. Studies show, however, that these commercially-raised animals pose much greater health risks than traditionally-raised ones. For example, let's look at beef, since the average American consumes upwards of 60 pounds of beef each year.

Having grown up on a small farm where we always raised our own cows, beef was a regular and much-enjoyed staple on our dinner table. I still remember the laughter and camaraderie in the kitchen as my family would gather to prepare meals together in the kitchen. The tantalizing aromas of onions and hamburger on the stove set the foundation for many a recipe. To this day, I either raise my own beef or purchase from a local farmer who raises grass-fed pastured beef. One thing I don't ever remember doing was draining off excessive fat from the meat after cooking. After years of home-grown beef, I was visiting a friend who had invited me and my family for dinner. She had purchased a couple pounds of hamburger from the local box store and had just started cooking it when we arrived. I was shocked at how much different this hamburger looked and smelled while it was cooking and how much grease it produced! Here are a few major differences between grass-fed beef and commercial beef:

- Commercial beef is generally raised on a diet rich in corn and other grains the second phase of their lives. Growers do this to boost growth. However, cows naturally are grass-eaters and thrive on a grass-only diet. Grain-fed beef has been proven to be higher in saturated fat.

- Commercial beef are often given hormones and other drugs to increase their growth in a shorter period of time. These "supplements" have been linked to an increased risk of cancer, pre-mature puberty, and infertility.
- Commercial beef are also on average given higher amounts of antibiotics, which can carry over into the meat. Crowded growing conditions and an often less sanitary environment increase the risk of illness, so many farmers will give antibiotics regularly.
- Conversely, grass-fed beef tends to have a healthier fatty acid composition and less total fat, twice as much Omega-3, contains higher amounts of essential minerals, antioxidants, and vitamins, and contain fewer toxic heavy metals, carcinogens, antibiotics, vaccines, and hormones. (*40) Plus, it just downright tastes better!

Similar examples could be given for the commercial poultry industry as well. When I was a kid, I remember raising chickens for eggs and for meat, and we never had different breeds for each. When my husband and I moved onto our homestead, I looked into raising chickens again for eggs and meat. I was shocked to learn about "meat birds" versus "egg layers" when purchasing chicks. The meat birds, I was told, were hybridized to go from incubator to freezer in just 8 weeks! Bred to grow unnaturally quickly, these chickens are what you get whenever you eat chicken from the grocery store or at a restaurant. But once again we see where man's attempts at improving on what God designed is backfiring on us. Although it may be better in terms of profit, what are the true implications of such a drastic genetic change on our health? How do they get a chicken to grow from egg to maturity in such a short time? The truth is, these birds have been genetically bred to have much higher estrogen levels, stimulating fast growth. The unfortunate side-effect, however, is that the high estrogen levels are then transferred through the meat to the consumer. Is it not a wonder then that we are seeing a rise in estrogen dominant related health issues such as young girls (and sometimes boys) developing breasts at ages as young as 8 or 9, puberty at younger ages, hormonal imbalances, and a rise in cases of breast cancer?

Even though the unit cost may seem a bit higher at the grocery store for an organically raised, animal with old-world genetics (although it's actually often a savings when you buy direct from the farmer...and sometimes that's the only place you can find it), the value is so much higher and worth the difference in terms of health benefits, taste, and peace of mind.

AND GOD SAID:

Romans 14: 21

It is better not to eat meat or drink wine or to do anything else that will cause your brother or sister to fall.

99

Exodus 12: 8

That same night they are to eat the meat roasted over the fire, along with bitter herbs, and bread made without yeast.

Mistake #4: Eating excessive processed meats that have chemical additives or other unhealthy ingredients added.

In our modern world where we desire foods that are convenient, efficient, and economical, the unfortunate result is the tendency to all too often turn to processed meats. Processed meats are those that have been preserved by curing, salting, drying, or canning, and include common choices such as sandwich meat, hot dogs, pepperoni, sausages, ham, canned meats, and most commercial jerky. The problem with many of these processed meats, even if we eliminate those made with pork, still are unhealthy and are linked with many health problems such as high blood pressure, heart disease, COPD (Chronic Obstructive Pulmonary Disease), diabetes, and several cancers including bowel and stomach cancer. (*41)

Processed meats often contain chemical additives such as binders and fillers, unhealthy refined salts, refined sugars, and proven cancer-causing substances like nitrites and nitrates. Sodium nitrite is added to many processed meats as a preservative, as a colorant, and as a flavor enhancer, but the unfortunate truth is sodium nitrite has been shown to increase the risk of cancer, particularly when the meat is heated above 265 degrees F (as is the case with most meats). In fact, in 2015, the World Health Organization classified processed meats as "Group 1 Carcinogens." Other Group 1 Carcinogens include tobacco and asbestos. (*42)

Generally, when I talk about avoiding processed meats, I get a lot of resistance. I understand. Really, I do. Having grown up on hot dogs, turkey sandwiches, and pepperoni pizza, the thought of avoiding these foods seemed crazy. But could these foods be part of the contributing factors why I had the health problems I did... the trouble sleeping, the weight gain, the skin issues, and the lack of energy? Changing the way you look at many of the foods you are accustomed to regularly consuming, can take some getting used to. Consider this, however. How much "light energy" is there in any processed meat? As we've discussed previously, the foods God directs us toward contains the most "light energy" either through direct or indirect absorption. Processed meats are dead foods. Very little "light energy" remains. The elements found in these meats are counter-productive, meaning they interfere with health and energy rather than give you health and energy.

Just because cultural norms and clever marketing have created an illusion that these foods are fine, doesn't make it so. Beware the wolves in sheep's clothing and turn your eyes to God's plan for your health.

When I first learned these concepts and started changing my habits, I was skeptical and resistant; and my husband even more so. As he often says, though, "the proof is in the pudding", and I was amazed at how much better I felt in a very short period of time when I shifted a few simple things in my menu planning and diet. God didn't say these things in the Bible for His benefit and He didn't say them for no reason. Don't take my word for it. Listen to what God is telling you about what is best for you and your family, then try it for yourself and experience the difference, too.

A Note About Bitter Herbs and Meat

In Exodus 12:8, scripture mentions including bitter herbs along with the meat consumed. Bitter herbs include parsley, kale, cilantro, basil, horseradish, arugula, dandelion leaves, peppermint, and chamomile, to name a few. Bitter herbs serve an important purpose in our diet, particularly when eating meat. Consuming bitter herbs stimulates the brain to release certain digestive hormones and enzymes. These hormones and enzymes are particularly important to digestion in that they stimulate the liver to increase the flow of bile, regulate the secretion of pancreatic hormones that regulate blood sugar, insulin, and glucagon, stimulate mechanisms to repair the gut wall, and stimulate the stomach muscles to prevent acid reflux.

When I was a kid, every plate included a sprig of parsley when we would eat at a restaurant. This parsley wasn't there for garnish, although it did serve that purpose as well. Rather, the parsley was meant to be consumed with the meat as a bitter herb to aide in digestion. Unfortunately, this tradition has long since been eliminated, much to the detriment of our gastric comfort. Other excellent bitter herbs include dandelion, mint, coriander, chicory, and endive.

Other benefits of bitter herbs include:
- Helping in the absorption of nutrients.
- Balancing the taste buds and controls sweet cravings.
- Helping the body cleansing of toxins.
- Stimulating metabolism.
- Fighting free radicals and stimulating the immune system.

AND GOD SAID:

Judges 6: 19

Gideon went inside, prepared a young goat, and from an ephah of flour he made bread without yeast. Putting the meat in a basket and its broth in a pot, he brought them out and offered them to him under the oak.

AND GOD SAID:

Adding some "bitters" to any meal with meat makes a significant enough difference that it bears mentioning and encouraging. Commercial bitters like "Swedish Bitters" are available, or simply add some parsley back onto your plate. Feel the difference for yourself.

Bone Broth

A powerful super-food that is often overlooked when formulating a healthy diet is bone broth. Broth is made by slow cooking the bones of "clean" animals in water with various vegetables and herbs. It is super easy and economical to make and is loaded with nutrients that support health and healing. Both science and folk tradition support the truth of the nutritional benefits of bone broth. Specific nutritional value will vary greatly depending on how the broth was made, including bones used, diet and nutrition of the animal, cooking methods, and other ingredients used. However, "bone broth, with its rich dissolves of collagen, cartilage, bone, and marrow, gives the body 'the right stuff' to rebuild and rejuvenate. These components also include vitamins and minerals, the conditionally essential amino acids glycine, proline, and glutamine, and healing 'essential' sugars knows as proteoglycans." (*43)

What exactly does that mean? Well, broth, when consumed regularly, "can give our bones strength and flexibility, our joints cushion and resilience, and our skin a youthful plumpness. What's more, the abundance of collagen in all types of bone broth supports heart health through strong and supple arteries, our vision with healthy corneas, digestion through gut healing, and overall disease prevention via immune system modulation... Broth even contributes to emotional stability and a positive mental attitude." (*43)

There's an old saying when you're sick with a cold or the flu to, "have some chicken soup, and call me in the morning." This old saying came from hundreds of years of country doctors (and grandmothers) who understood the healing power of bone broth, and prescribed it to their patients. They may not have understood the science behind *why* broth was so effective at healing; they just knew it worked. So much so, that a popular modern-day publishing company created a whole series on "Chicken Soup for the Soul" which consisted of a compilation of stories and anecdotes to help "heal" our soul.

For your convenience, we have included super simple instructions on how to make your own broth in our "Recipes" section under "Nourishing Broth." If you are interested in more detailed information about broth, you can find an entire online tutorial in our Living Foods Academy found at **www.HealthyHomesteadLiving.com**. If you choose to purchase commercially made broth rather than make your own, be sure to read the labels and stick with versions that don't use MSG, refined table salt, or other chemical additives. Commercial broth won't have as much collagen or gelatin in them, which are the key components that give broth the powerful healing, so whenever possible, I encourage you to make your own.

Eggs

Eggs are not often mentioned in the Bible, but the few references we do find, including Job 6:6 and Luke 11:12 are clear that eggs were an accepted part of the biblical table. Eggs, despite some controversy over the years about cholesterol, are a healthy addition to your diet and can be consumed regularly. Be sure to choose organic, free-range eggs whenever possible, as those eggs have been proven to be higher in nutrients, a better source of protein, and lower in cholesterol than commercially raised eggs. Although chicken eggs tend to be the most common, any egg from a "clean" bird can be enjoyed such as duck eggs, quail eggs, and turkey eggs.

Spiritual Significance of Meat

Particularly in the Old Testament, meat held great spiritual significance as an offering to God. God's people carefully considered the sacrifice the animal was making, and not something that was taken for granted. Each sacrifice had a specific purpose, such as offering thanksgiving, as an atonement for a sin, or as a celebration commemorating a holy day.

> *"Those offering a sacrifice felt that they were giving up something from their prized possessions. People owned animals as sources of labor or food, as well as a form of capital; hence slaughtering them in connection with the Temple rites was a sacrifice of a precious source of income and food.*
>
> *The animal was not considered just a distant commodity as is generally the case in today's world of corporate agriculture; rather, it was a creature that the owner raised and saw on a daily basis, and whose needs were a matter of personal responsibility and even concern...*

AND GOD SAID:

Isaiah 55: 2

Listen carefully to Me, and eat what is good, and delight yourself in abundance.

The emotional result on the one who brought the sacrifice and watched it being killed was to contemplate that because of their sin they deserved to be the ones on the altar. Thus they would experience feelings of repentance and become transformed, worthy of a renewed lease on life." (*44)

Jesus, having died on the cross as the ultimate sacrifice, washed away our sins, negating the need for us to continue the traditions of the Old Testament in sacrificing animals for our sins. When eating meat, it would still behoove us to reverently consider and appreciate the life that was given so that we may eat that meat, which offers us energy. Too often in our modern society we become disassociated with much of where our food comes from.

My mom used to tell a story about when I was about 3 or 4 years old. We raised our own beef, and that year we had a black Angus steer that I had named "Macaroni." Even though I was so little, I do remember helping feed Macaroni and brushing his coat sometimes. My grandmother, as the story goes, came to visit some months later and we were having hamburgers for dinner. Over dinner, I turned to my mom and innocently asked, "Is this Macaroni?" My grandmother turned to me and patting my hand, said, "No, sweetie, this is hamburger." Sheepishly, my mom had to confirm to my poor grandma that, "Actually, yes. This is Macaroni." For years my mom would laugh about this story and the priceless look on my grandmother's face.

I can say from personal experience that when you have a deep personal experience raising animals for food, that you develop a rich appreciation for that animal, the work that goes into raising the animal, and the sacrifice that is made so that we may live and thrive.

Jesus made the ultimate sacrifice so that through His blood, we may be washed of our sins. I encourage you to not take for granted the sacrifice made by the animal when you eat meat, nor the sacrifice Jesus made for you so that you may be forgiven of all your sins, washed clean by His blood.

Chapter Summary:

Including meat in your diet is perfectly acceptable in the eyes of God, according to His directives in both the Old and New Testament, however when making choices of what to include on your plate, it is important to only consume "clean" meat. In addition to only eating clean meat, it is also important to keep portion size within a healthy range and to avoid gluttony. Meat can offer nutritional benefits for health, including essential amino acids, proteins, and enzymes; yet not all meat is created equal. Choose wisely for optimum benefits.

Action Steps:

1. Eliminate any unclean meats from your diet, replacing them with those meats God defines as clean and acceptable.
2. Reduce portion size, if necessary, keeping each meal to 4-6 ounces or less of meat (about the size of the palm of your hand).
3. Purchase only meat that has been raised and processed in ways that is closest to God's original design. For example, opt for grass-feed beef or bison and free-range, organic foundation-bred poultry. Although the prices may be a bit higher, they are worth the extra expense for the increased nutritional value and benefits to your health.
4. Avoid processed meats, particularly those with a long list of ingredients you can't pronounce.
5. Add some bitter herbs to your dish when consuming meats.
6. Try consuming some bone broth in soups, stews, sauces, or condiments at least a couple times a week to get the incredible healing benefits of this powerful superfood.
7. Always pray over your food, and when eating meat, prayerfully offer a word of thanksgiving to the sacrifices made for your nourishment.

Theologenic Diet
List of Clean Meats

The following is a summary of meats you can enjoy as discussed in this chapter. This list is by no means complete, yet is meant as a basic guideline to get you started and show you the diversity of healthy options available. This list is courtesy of "What the Bible Teaches about Clean and Unclean Meats", page 19-21 (*39).

Mammals that chew the cud and have split hooves:
Antelope
Bison (buffalo)
Caribou
Cattle (beef, veal)
Deer (venison)
Elk
Gazelle
Giraffe
Goat (chevron)
Moose
Ox
Reindeer
Sheep (lamb, mutton)

Fish with fins and scales:
Anchovy
Bass
Bluefish
Bluegill
Carp
Cod
Crappie
Drum
Flounder
Grouper
Grunt
Haddock
Hake
Halibut
Hardhead
Herring (or alewife)
Kingfish
Mackerel (or cobia)
Minnow
Mullet
Perch (or bream)
Pike (or pickerel or jack)
Pollack (or pollock or Boston bluefish)
Rockfish
Salmon
Sardine (or pilchard)
Shad
Silver hake (or whiting)

Smelt (or frost fish or ice fish)
Snapper
Sole
Steelhead
Sucker
Sunfish
Tarpon
Trout (or weakfish)
Tuna
Turbot
Whitefish

Birds with clean characteristics:
Chicken
Dove
Duck
Goose
Grouse
Guinea fowl
Partridge
Peafowl
Pheasant
Pigeon
Prairie chicken
Quail
Sage-hen
Sparrow (and other songbirds)
Swan
Turkey

Insects:
Locusts
Crickets
Grasshoppers

Bone Broth made from the bones of clean animals.
Beef broth
Chicken broth
Fish broth
Turkey broth

Eggs from Free-Range Clean Birds

Theologenic Diet
List of Unclean Meats

The following is a summary of meats God defines as unclean and should be **avoided**. These meats tend to carry more diseases, toxins, and parasites while offering little nutritional benefit in relation to the potential harmful side-effects.

Swine:
Boar
Peccary
Pig (hog, bacon, ham,
 lard, pork, most
 sausage and
 Pepperoni)

Canines:
Coyote
Dog
Fox
Hyena
Jackal
Wolf

Felines:
Cat
Cheetah
Leopard
Lion
Panther
Tiger

Equines:
Donkey (ass)
Horse
Mule
Onager
Zebra (quagga)

Other Unclean Land Animals:
Armadillo
Badger
Bat
Bear
Beaver
Camel
Elephant
Gorilla
Groundhog

Hippopotamus
Kangaroo
Llama (alpaca, vicuña)
Mole
Monkey
Mouse
Muskrat
Opossum
Porcupine
Rabbit (hare)
Raccoon
Rat
Rhinoceros
Skunk
Slug
Snail (escargot)
Squirrel
Wallaby
Weasel
Wolverine
Worm

All insects except those in the locust family.

Reptiles:
Alligator
Caiman
Crocodile
Lizard
Snake
Turtle

Amphibians:
Blindworm
Frog
Newt
Salamander
Toad

Unclean meats, continued:

Marine animals without fins and scales:
Bullhead
Catfish
Eel
European turbot
Marlin
Paddlefish
Shark
Stickleback
Squid
Sturgeon (includes most caviar)
Swordfish

Shellfish:
Abalone
Clam
Conch
Crab
Crayfish (crawfish, crawdad)
Lobster
Mussel
Oyster
Scallop
Shrimp (prawn)

Soft body:
Cuttlefish
Jellyfish
Limpet
Octopus
Squid (calamari)

Sea mammals:
Dolphin
Otter
Porpoise
Seal
Walrus
Whale

Birds of prey, scavengers, and others:
Albatross
Bittern
Buzzard
Condor
Coot
Cormorant
Crane
Crow
Cuckoo
Eagle
Flamingo
Grebe
Grosbeak
Gull
Hawk
Heron
Kite
Lapwing
Loon
Magpie
Osprey
Ostrich
Owl
Parrot
Pelican
Penguin
Plover
Rail
Raven
Roadrunner
Sandpiper
Seagull
Stork
Swallow
Swift
Vulture
Water hen
Woodpecker

Notes:

Chapter 8: The Truth About Dairy

Physical Significance of Dairy

Milk, it does the body good....right? Well, yes and no. This well-known marketing slogan created by the dairy industry doesn't tell the whole story. Neither does the other popular marketing slogan, "Got Milk?" Scriptures mention milk many times, and it is clear that people during biblical times consumed dairy regularly. In fact, Abraham gave milk to visiting angels as described in Genesis 18:8.

The milk of the Bible was much different than the milk most of you may be grabbing out of your refrigerator to enjoy with a plate of cookies. Let's take a quick look at a few major differences and what you need to know about consuming dairy to maximize the health benefits...or potential problems to your health.

Modern Dairy vs. Traditional Dairy

When the Israelites were led out of Egypt during the Exodus, they were given a land "flowing with milk and honey." Dairy, in one form or another, is mentioned close to 100 times in the Bible. It is clear that God's original intention was for milk to be a healthy addition to our diet. However, the topic of milk has become one of the most controversial in the health-food industry today with arguments that milk is unhealthy and should be avoided. In the case of modern commercial milk, I would agree. Modern commercial milk tends to be acidifying to the body, be mucous-producing, contain antibiotics and growth hormones, and an imbalance of vitamins (which I will explain further later in this chapter). Milk, as most of you are consuming it, is not the milk of scripture.

This doesn't mean you have to give up milk altogether. You can still enjoy milk and diary products by simply making a few adjustment to the type of milk and dairy you are buying. Truth be told, milk has the potential of being a powerful superfood that offers a vast array of nutrients to support health. The difference between toxic milk and healthy milk can be found in the genetics of the animal, how the animal was raised, what the animal ate, how the milk was handled/processed, and how you consume it.

Most commercial diary, much like the commercial meat industries, has developed a system based on efficiency and maximizing profits. Our love affair with diary

AND GOD SAID:

Genesis 18: 8

And he took butter, and milk, and the calf which he had dressed, and set it before them; and he stood by them under the tree, and they did eat.

Leviticus 20: 24

But I have said unto you, Ye shall inherit their land, and I will give it unto you to possess it, a land that floweth with milk and honey; I am the Lord you God, which have separated you from other people. (NKJV)

products, particularly milk, butter, ice cream, and cheese, has driven commercial dairy operations to make significant changes over the years that hasn't always resulted in a better end product. In some cases, not only is taste sacrificed, but health benefits as well. Here are a few important things to consider when choosing which dairy products to purchase and consume:

Genetics of the Animal:

Milk is made up of about 85% water, with the remaining 15% comprised of vitamins, minerals, fat, carbohydrates (lactose), and protein. The lactose, or milk sugar, is often blamed when someone has a reaction to drinking milk. This is because people who have a low tolerance to milk may lack intestinal *lactase*, an enzyme that digests lactose. All baby mammals produce lactase, but production declines after weaning, depending on the genetics of the mammal. In humans, an estimated 30-40% of the world's population produces lactase into adulthood, and those who don't can still generally tolerate consuming milk products in small quantities without problems. In most cases, the lactose is not what is causing the intolerance or reaction; rather it is more likely the milk casein causing trouble in the body. (*45)

Protein in milk is about 20% whey protein and about 80% casein. Casein is the part of the milk that is the most difficult to digest, and the assimilation and digestibility of the milk depends on the type of casein produced by the animal. Casein proteins can be divided into three types: alpha-, beta-, and kappa-casein. The beta-casein can then further be classified as Beta-Casein A1 or A2, with their primary differences being their amino acid structure. Human milk, as well as most goat milk and most sheep milk, is predominantly beta-casein A2 type and generally is more easily digested than A1 beta-casein.

A1 beta-casein, which is found in about 99% of commercial cow's milk in America, affects the body a little differently. When A1 beta-casein is consumed, the body creates a small fragment of protein called beta-casomorphin 7 (or BCM7). *(I know we're getting a little scientific and technical here, but stay with me a sec as this may be a huge moment of enlightenment for you like it was for me when I first learned it, and help you understand why milk is so controversial on its health benefits.)*

BCM7 has been shown in numerous clinical studies to cause inflammation in the body, and has been linked to minor irritations such as bloating, cramps, gas, and diarrhea, as well as more chronic and serious issues such as diabetes, cancer, IBS, heart disease, autism, and Alzheimer's, among others! (*46) Therefore, consuming milk with A1 beta-casein may not be the best choice, particularly if you are suffering from any health issues, especially chronic ones. Some recent studies on the effects of BCM7 on the body are going so far as to say that A1 beta-casein consumption may be even more harmful to the body than gluten. Where gluten intolerance affects two receptor sites in your gut, BCM7 can affect up to twenty-six receptor sites! (*47)

> *"The body recognizes BCM7 as a foreign protein and launches an attack by the immune system. If you've ever wondered why you feel increased phlegm in your lungs or digestive tract after consuming a dairy product, it could be the presence of BCM7, which selectively binds to the epithelial cells in mucous membranes and stimulates mucus production... Depending on the genetic makeup of the person, the body can become susceptible to illnesses like Type 1 diabetes, neurological impairments such as autism and schizophrenia, impaired immune function, autoimmune diseases, and heart disease, as well as joint and muscle pains, fatigue, digestive disturbances, and headaches." (*47, page 161)*

A1 beta-casein milk is found in most commercial breeds of cows, particularly European and American breeds, most notably Holsteins. A2 beta-casein is found in older breeds of cows from Africa, India, and the Middle East, most goat breeds, and most sheep breeds. Choosing milk that genetically produces A2 beta-casein will more closely follow God's original intent for milk as a healthy addition to the diet. By simply switching to milk that your body more naturally can absorb and digest, you can enjoy all those delicious dairy favorites without the adverse reactions. Granted, finding A2 beta-casein milk in your area may be a bit tricky since you typically won't find it at your local grocery store. Organic goat milk is one option that is more readily available, or you can search online to find a local dairy in your area who might have fresh A2 beta-casein milk. Look for milk from Guernsey, Jersey, or Fleckvieh breeds. Although they can still contain A1, these breeds have a higher incidence of A2 genetics. Many local dairy farmers will have DNA tests that will show what kind of milk their stock is producing.

For more detailed information about the science behind A1 versus A2 beta-casein milk, read *Devil in the Milk* by Keith Woodford. This book goes into much more detail about the differences, how they affect the body, and how some specialists are linking A1 beta-casein milk to major health issues today.

AND GOD SAID:

Deuteronomy 32: 13-14

He nourished him with honey from the rock, and with oil from the flinty crag, with curds and milk from the herd and flock, and with fattened lambs and goats... (NIV)

Proverbs 27: 27

And thou shalt have goats' milk enough for thy food, for the food of thy household, and for the maintenance for thy servants. (KJV)

I realize that this may be a drastic change for you, and if it is too extreme a shift for you right now, that's ok. Before making any major changes such as where you buy your milk or the type of diary you consume, try going off dairy for a short time (2-3 weeks) and see if you can tell a difference in how you feel, particularly muscle aches, fatigue, mucous, allergies, ear infections, and digestive issues. If you see improvement, you may consider eliminating dairy or slowly adding A2 beta-casein back into your diet while monitoring your body's reactions.

I grew up in Wisconsin, in the heart of dairy country. Almost everyone I knew either lived on or worked on a dairy farm. Dairy, particularly milk, butter, ice cream, and cheese, were included in almost every meal in one way or another. To this day I have a particular affinity for cheese! As a child, I don't ever remember having any reactions to consuming dairy, but as I got older I found that those age-old favorites, particularly milk, didn't quite agree with me like they used to. When my daughter was a toddler, she would react severely to any commercial milk, with painful rashes and skin breakouts. We found that she did fine on goat milk, and thrived on cultured dairy products like kefir and yogurt. After learning about the differences between A1 and A2 beta-casein in the milk, I could more fully understand why we were both experiencing reactions as our bodies were trying to deal with the BCM7 produced. Since switching to A2 beta-casein diary products as our primary choices, we both have a renewed enjoyment in consuming our favorite dairy products without the health issues previously experienced.

How the dairy animal was raised:

Other than the genetics behind the dairy product, it is also important to consider the management practices behind the animal producing your dairy. As with beef, there is significant scientific evidence that grass-fed/pasture-raised diary is much healthier than grain-fed dairy.

Grass-fed cattle produce milk that is higher in alpha-linolenic acid (ALA), which is an omega-3 fat that has been shown to help reduce inflammation in the body. In some studies, grass-fed milk showed double the omega-3 fat content as milk from conventionally-raised dairy cows. Data also shows grass-fed milk to be higher in selenium, vitamin B12, vitamin E, calcium, beta-carotene, and conjugated linoleic acid (CLA), a fatty acid that has been found to be beneficial in reducing the risk of certain cancers and heart disease. (*48)

The vitamin content of the milk is an important aspect that is often overlooked. Consider this. The United States is the number one milk-drinking nation on the planet; yet also the number one in incidences of osteoporosis. For years, we've been told by the dairy industry to drink milk for the calcium for strong bones. Why, then, would we have such a problem with osteoporosis, a condition where the bones become brittle and fragile? To understand this question we have to look at how the body works. Vitamins often don't work by themselves in supporting the body. Instead, they work in conjunction with each other. In the case of milk, there may be calcium but there is not enough magnesium, boron, copper, zinc, and vitamin C, which are equally important for optimal bone support. Additionally, milk contains phosphorous, which is also important for bone development, but in such high levels that it actually *decreases* the calcium availability to the body. Dr. Linda Folden Palmer, in her book *Baby Matters* further explains by saying:

> *"Decades of effort to demonstrate that high calcium diets chiefly derived from dairy products build strong bones have failed to prove any such correlation. In fact, the opposite seems to be true... A balanced intake of all the bone minerals, [boron, copper, zinc, magnesium, and calcium], along with adequate vitamin A, C, and D, is what is truly needed. A balanced intake of minerals cannot occur when the diet emphasizes dairy. Dairy's high calcium causes relative deficiencies in magnesium and other bone-building minerals, and its high phosphorus and animal protein reduces calcium availability... Vegetable sources are superior to dairy for calcium and other nutrients in many ways. (*49, page 265)*

If you are drinking milk under the misconception that it is needed solely for the calcium, particularly in the case of our children, you might want to reconsider. Hopefully these facts clear that up for you. Additionally, many brands of milk in small cartons, such as those served in most schools, not only come from A1 beta-casein cows, but also have sugar and other flavor enhancing ingredients added.

If that isn't enough to convince you to reevaluate your milk, consider also that commercially raised dairy cows tend to get higher incidences of antibiotics and growth hormones to stimulate milk production. These drugs are then transferred to the milk. One growth hormone in particular, Recombinant Bovine Growth Hormone (rBGH), should be avoided. rBGH was first introduced in 1993 after its approval by the Food and Drug Administration, and has become a popular "supplement" in commercial dairy due to its ability to increase milk production. Although this GMO product created by Monsanto does its job of increasing profits

AND GOD SAID:

Judges 5: 25

He asked for water, and she gave him milk; she brought forth butter in a lordly dish. (KJV)

Isaiah 7: 22

And because of the abundance of the milk produced he will eat curds, for everyone that is left within the land will eat curds and honey. (NASB)

for the dairy industry, studies are showing that consumption of rBGH milk increases the risk of lung cancer, colon cancer, breast cancer, prostate cancer, and uterine cancer. Other studies hypothesize that the rBGH in the milk is the primary culprit for adolescent girls developing breasts and starting their cycles at increasingly younger ages. This growth hormone has been banned in many international communities, yet is still being used in the United States. Look for milk that is labeled rBGH/rBST free.

How the dairy products are consumed:

People in biblical times had no refrigeration to keep their dairy products nice and chilled like we do today. Most of the time, if not consuming fresh, raw milk right from the animal (most often from goats or sheep), they enjoyed dairy in the form of butter, cheese, or cultured products like clabbered milk, kefir, or yogurt. In fact, some scrolls found in Turkey from Abraham referenced fermented milk products as one of the keys to his long and healthy life. (*50)

Cultured dairy, or fermented dairy, is simply using naturally occurring good bacteria to preserve the milk. During fermentation, the bacteria ingest the lactose and break down some of the casein, making the end product much more digestible and filled with beneficial probiotic (good) bacteria that benefit the gut. Even people who experience reactions to commercial milk, often find they can enjoy cultured dairy without the adverse effects.

Cultured dairy is versatile, delicious, and easy to make. And with health benefits such as reducing constipation, reducing seasonal allergies, enhancing digestion, encouraging deep sleep, and immune system support, cultured dairy is a worthwhile way to enjoy your dairy. Some of our favorite cultured dairy choices include kefir (the most potent with upwards of 35 different strains of beneficial probiotics), yogurt, cultured sour cream, cultured butter (and the delicious cultured buttermilk, which you get when you make your own butter), and kefir ice cream.

Check out the recipe section in this book for simple instructions on how to make your own kefir and yogurt. When buying commercial versions, look for organic A2 options whenever possible, and avoid any versions that are flavored, as they often have too much sugar added. Plain, unsweetened varieties can easily be flavored with your favorite fruit, herbs, essential oils, or spices, and they also tend to work better when using as an ingredient in recipes.

Pasteurized, Homogenized, or Raw?

No discussion about milk and the differences between healthy dairy and unhealthy dairy would be complete without addressing the differences between pasteurized and homogenized milk versus raw milk. Again we enter a much debated and controversial topic, yet one that bears addressing. Most commercial dairy is both pasteurized and homogenized, but what exactly does that mean and how does it affect the milk?

Pasteurization was discovered by Louis Pasteur in 1856 when he was commissioned by an alcohol manufacturer to discover a way to avoid their wine from turning sour. In his research, he discovered that the grape juice was turned into wine by a certain strain of yeast; but the soured wine also contained another organism which more closely resembled the bacteria found in vinegar. Through his experiments, he discovered that by heating the wine to a certain temperature, the wine had a lesser likelihood of the vinegar bacteria growing out of hand and contaminating the batch. It wasn't until the late 1800's that his research was applied to milk, in an attempt to reduce the cases of tuberculosis. Although cases of tuberculosis did decline, it took several decades for pasteurized milk to really start becoming mainstream, and this success was mostly due to political lobbying rather than consumer demand.

Pasteurization involves heating the milk to a temperature between 161.6°F to 165.2°F (72°C to 74°C) for a period of 15 to 30 seconds. Ultra-pasteurization takes the milk to even higher temperatures between 275°F and 284°F (135°C to 140°C) for 3 to 5 seconds. This heating process does destroy potentially harmful bacteria that may be in the milk, however, it also does several other things including the following:
- It denatures natural enzymes in the milk.
- It destroys some of the vitamins and minerals.
- It decreases the bio availability of folic acid and other nutrients found in the milk.
- It alters the proteins in the milk, changing how the milk acts when used to make other foods like yogurt, cheese, and cultured dairy.
- It causes a chemical reaction between proteins and sugars, causing yellowing or discoloration of the milk.

In a nutshell, pasteurization destroys both the good and the bad bacteria in the milk, but it also changes the molecular structure of the milk making it less

AND GOD SAID:

Proverbs 30:33

Surely the churning of milk bringeth forth butter, and the wringing of the nose bringeth forth blood. (KJV)

Isaiah 7: 15

Butter and honey shall he eat, that he may know to refuse the evil, and choose the good. (KJV)

palatable and less healthy.   In order to make this pasteurized milk more appealing to the consumer, in most cases milk is then homogenized.

Homogenization is the process in which the milk is highly pressurized, which essentially breaks down the fat globules so that they stay dispersed in the milk rather than emulsifying and rising to the top. Although this process results in a more aesthetic milk, it also has been shown to:
- Oxidize milk fats making them more carcinogenic and toxic to the body.
- Release the enzyme Xanthine Oxidase, which has been shown to adhere to arterial walls and contribute to heart disease.
- Alter the fat molecule so that the body often recognizes them as antigens, stimulating an immune response. (*51)

All too often, man thinks he can do better than God, but God's design is always perfect. As stated in Proverbs 30: 33, the churning of milk should bring forth butter. When we alter the milk through homogenization, the milk no longer brings forth butter and therefore it no longer follows God's plan. It's not surprising then that the health benefits are no longer there. We have once again taken a living food, filled with life energy, and made it into a dead food, devoid of benefits.

But, you may ask, what about raw milk? Isn't it unsafe? What about the problem of potentially getting sick if I don't drink pasteurized milk? Well, those are great questions and I'm so glad you asked! Raw milk has been a staple food for many cultures for thousands of years. Keep in mind that the science of pasteurization is a pretty recent development; and one that arose out of a need created by the growing commercial dairy industry. Modern dairies have no choice but to collect the milk from hundreds of cows at one time, pooling their milk into large vats. Any contaminated milk from either a sick cow or possible contaminated equipment is mixed with all the other milk. Even though this may be a rare occurrence, by default the need exists as a precautionary measure. As a result, the need to treat all the milk becomes necessary. Raw milk from one of these facilities would most likely be considered unsafe and not recommended.

However, if the cow, goat, sheep, or other mammal is healthy and monitored closely for potential illness or disease, fed quality forage, allowed to enjoy sunshine, and the milk is collected using sanitary practices, the likelihood of the milk containing harmful pathogens is pretty slim. Most small dairy farms are meticulous in their attention to detail on the health of their animals and the quality of the product they produce. I know many dairy farmers and have visited countless farms both cow and goat and I always find it educational and inspiring. The dedicated men and women who choose dairy farming as their profession have a true love for their animals, and it often shows when you see them interacting with their stock. And, it's especially heart-warming to see their animals respond in kind.

Consuming raw milk from a clean facility with healthy animals is not only safe, but the milk is in a form that contains the highest possible nutritional value over the processed alternatives.

Consider the difference:

1. A1 beta-casein milk that has been ultra-pasteurized and homogenized, then transported to your grocery store in plastic containers.
2. A2 beta-casein raw organic milk from grass-fed animals, stored in glass jars.

Now that we have discussed the differences, you can see why milk has become such a controversial topic when discussing health. The two choices may look the same, be called the same thing, and appear to be the same, but you are comparing apples to oranges. Option 1, which is what you most commonly find commercially and the milk most people are used to consuming, is harmful to the point of being toxic. Option 2, describes the milk of the Bible. Milk and dairy products that are wholesome, full of nutrients, and beneficial to the body.

Note: Recent legislation has prohibited the sale of raw milk in many areas of the country. If you live in one of those areas, contact your local legislative offices to have your voice heard. Even in areas where raw milk is prohibited from commercial sale, you can often find a local farmer and purchase your milk directly from them.

Also, any time I refer to milk in this chapter, I am referring to whole milk only. Reduced fat milk, 1%, 2%, or skim are all highly processed milks and lack the nutritional value of whole milk.

AND GOD SAID:

Hebrews 5: 12-14

Though by this time you ought to be teachers, you need someone to teach you the elementary truths of God's word all over again. You need milk, not solid food! Anyone who lives on milk, being still an infant, is not acquiainted with the teaching about righteousness. But solid food is for the mature, who by constant use have trained themselves to distinguish good from evil.

1 Corinthians 3: 2

I gave you milk, not solid food, for you were not ready. Even now you are not yet ready... (NIV)

A Word About Alternative Milks

Alternative milks are rising in popularity and for good reason. With most commercial milk being of the A1 beta-casein pasteurized and homogenized variety, health-conscious individuals are looking for better options. Alternative milk choices include increasingly popular selections like almond milk, coconut milk, and soy milk. For best results, select varieties that have minimal processing and no chemical or sugar additives.

Almond milk is easy to make yourself, making it my personal favorite, as it is economical, nutritious, and full of flavor when made at home. I have included instructions in the recipe section if you are interested in trying this easy milk alternative yourself. My daughter had a sleep-over with some friends one time and for fun we did a blind, side-by-side, taste-test of my homemade almond milk and some organic store-bought almond milk. Hands down, the homemade almond milk won for better flavor. Many of the girls even preferred it over cow's milk. With a good blender, almond milk takes less than 5 minutes to make and is a wonderful milk alternative. We especially love using it in our smoothies and in our pancakes.

When selecting soy milk, be sure to read the label carefully, as the majority of soy grown in the United States is now GMO and much less desirable if health is your main concern. Soy is another controversial topic in the health-food industry since there have been some studies linking soy to disrupting hormone levels, particularly estrogen. Reports on soy go both ways, so if you are a fan of soy, be sure to stick with organic, non-processed, non-GMO varieites.

Spiritual Significance of Milk

In the Old Testament, milk is often referred to together with honey, as in the "land of milk and honey." The general interpretation for the significance of milk and honey in these verses represents God' love for us and His desire to give us all things good, bountiful, and plentiful. Other interpretations reference milk as a symbol of fertility and abundance.

In the New Testament, milk takes on a much different spiritual meaning. As tiny babies, we are vulnerable and require special care. We are completely at the mercy of our caregivers for our well-being in every aspect of our lives including our food, our clothing, our comfort, and our sense of belonging and being loved.

When we are spiritually reborn through Christ we are just as we were as helpless babies, requiring special care to sustain us as we mature and grow to handle bigger and better. Initially, we receive our spiritual milk through the Word of God to sustain us as we grow. Paul alludes to this in his letter to Corinth when he says, "I fed you with milk, not solid food, for you were not ready for it. And even now you are not yet ready..." (1Cor. 3:2, ESV).

It is logical to look at milk as a symbol of our constant need for God's care, guidance, and involvement in our lives. Just as we turned to our mother or father when we were babies, we now turn to our Heavenly Father in our Christian walk. I am often humbled by His unfailing support when I turn to Him in prayer for all areas of my life.

AND GOD SAID:

1 Peter 2: 2-3

Like newborn babes, crave pure spiritual milk, so that by it you may grow up in your salvation, now that you have tasted that the Lord is Good.

Theologenic Diet
List of Dairy

The following is a summary of dairy you can enjoy as discussed in this chapter. This list is by no means complete, yet is meant as a basic guideline to get you started and show you the diversity of healthy options available. Choose dairy that is:

A2 Beta-Casein Organic, Grass-Fed Dairy

Amasi
Butter
Buttermilk
Cheddar Cheese
Cheese Curds
Colby Cheese
Colby-Jack Cheese
Clabber
Condensed Milk
Cottage Cheese
Cream Cheese
Crème Fraiche
Curds
Custard
Evaporated Milk
Farmer's Cheese
Ghee (clarified butter)
Greek Yogurt
Ice Cream (Homemade Best)
Kefir
Lassi
Monterey Jack Cheese
Mozzarella Cheese
Muenster Cheese
Pepper Jack Cheese
Powdered Milk
Provelone Cheese
Quark
Raw Whole Milk (Camel, Cow, Goat, Sheep)
Raw Heavy Cream
Ricotta Cheese
Sour Cream
String Cheese
Swiss Cheese
Whey
Whey Protein
Whipped Cream (Homemade Best)
Yogurt

Alternative Dairy:

Almond Milk
Almond Milk Kefir
Cashew Milk
Coconut Butter
Coconut Milk
Hemp Milk
Soy Milk (Organic, non-GMO only)

Chapter Summary:

Dairy can either be a highly nutritious or highly toxic part of your diet, depending on the type of dairy you consume and your body's ability to digest it. Assuming your body can handle dairy, only organic A2 beta-casein type dairy from grass-fed animals follow God's original design, offering the best health benefits. Some of the best dairy products are those that have been cultured or fermented, such as kefir and yogurt, as these products will support the immune system and the entire digestive tract via the beneficial probiotics found in them. Alternative dairy products, such as those made from almonds or coconuts, also represent viable options.

Action Steps:

1. Eliminate any and all commercial dairy products from your diet that come from A1 beta-casein genetics. Consider "fasting" from dairy altogether for a period of at least 2-3 weeks, and monitor how you feel when off dairy.
2. If you decide to resume dairy in your diet, choose only organic A2 beta-casein grass-fed dairy products or dairy alternatives.
3. Try to add some cultured dairy such as kefir and yogurt into your diet every day.
4. Prayerfully consider where you are in your walk with God. Are you still a baby, needing only spiritual milk, or have you progressed into more substance? What can you do to encourage your personal spiritual growth? This may be between you and God, or it may benefit you to join a study group or support group through a church, as spiritual growth can be better supported through collaboration.

Notes:

Chapter 9: Honey & Sweets

Physical Significance of Honey & Sweets

Since so many verses in Scripture link milk with honey, the next logical progression in our discussion is to talk about honey... and all her sweet cousins that we love so well. Of the five tastes our tongue recognizes (sweet, sour, salty, bitter, and umami or savory), none capture our interest and desires quite as much as sweet. Even just thinking the word "sweet" can bring a smile to our faces and uplift our spirits.

Interestingly, there are about 65 verses in the Bible that mention honey, depending on the translation, and 157 occurrences with a reference to "sweet", however not once does Scripture mention sugar or any other sweetener besides honey that I could find. There are references to sweet herbs, sweet spices, sweet milk, sweet incense, sweet oil, sweet smells, and sweet savour but fundamentally the only true sweetener God mentions is honey. Does this mean we shouldn't consume other sweeteners? Not necessarily, but when you look deeper into the science behind the primary sweeteners on the market, there are a few that stand out a full head and shoulders above the rest in terms of health benefits (and a few in terms of health detriments). Let's look at the facts about the top sweetener choices so you can make better decisions on which sweeteners are right for you and your health.

Honey

Of all the foods on the planet, I find honey to be one of the most fascinating. A study of honey truly demonstrates God's detailed artistry and the complexity of His creations. Honey comes from bees, but not just any bee. There are over 20,000 species of bees on the planet, but only 7 species of honeybees that produce this delicious ambrosia. Honeybees live in large colonies consisting of one queen, a few drones, and tens of thousands of worker bees. The queen and all the worker bees are female, each with a specific job that she does her whole life, and does well. To make honey, a worker bee collects nectar and pollen from various flowers (aiding in pollination in the process, responsible for an estimated 75% of the world's food crops). The nectar is then stored in one of the bee's two stomachs, which mixes the nectar with special enzymes. The bee then regurgitates this mixture, sometimes into the mouth of another bee, to mix with its saliva, before depositing it into the honeycomb to be dehydrated to the perfect

AND GOD SAID:

Proverbs 24: 13

My son, eat thou honey, because it is good; and the honeycomb, which is sweet to thy taste. (KJV)

Proverbs 16: 24

Gracious words are a honeycomb, sweet to the soul and healing to the bones. (NIV)

moisture level. Bees dehydrate the honey by rapidly fanning their wings to circulate air. Once the honey reaches the perfect consistency and moisture content, the bees cap off the honeycomb with beeswax which comes from a special gland in their abdomens, then collected by other bees and chewed.

In order to produce one pound of honey, an average of 60,000 honeybees must travel about 55,000 miles and visit approximately two million flowers. Each worker bee visits between 50 and 100 flowers during each collection flight and produces an average of 1/12 teaspoon of honey in her lifetime. The average bee colony produces between 60 and 100 pounds of honey each year. (*51)

When we consider how honey is made in conjunction with our goal to consume living foods with as much "life energy" as possible, honey ranks quite high. Bees make the honey directly from the pollen and nectar that the plants created from the sun's energy, then add their own special mix of enzymes and amino acids to form a truly unique and amazing substance!

Interestingly, honey can be stored pretty much indefinitely and does not spoil. Archaeological digs have unearthed honey that dates back thousands of years, and upon further testing, found the honey to still be good for consumption! Unlike almost all other "life energy" foods, honey has an almost unlimited shelf-life, while still retaining that powerful nutritional value.

Honey itself is comprised of a combination of water, glucose, fructose, over 20 other complex sugars, enzymes, vitamins, amino acids, and essential minerals like calcium, iron, magnesium, phosphate, and potassium. Honey is antibacterial, antiviral, antiseptic, anti-microbial, anti-fungal, anti-inflammatory, and antioxidant, and has been used for thousands of years as a medicine, a food, and a sweetener.

Medicinally, honey has been proven to help with burns, wounds, coughs, allergies, acid reflux, diarrhea, infections, stomach ulcers, high blood pressure, jaundice, eczema, inflammation, and arthritis. The antibacterial qualities have proven to be effective against dozens of harmful bacteria strains including E. Coli and salmonella while not jeopardizing the good bacteria in the digestive system. But, the best part is, it just simply tastes amazing!

One word of caution, however. It is generally recommended by healthcare professionals to not give honey to infants under one year old. Most specialists discourage babies consuming honey because the natural good bacteria in their stomachs haven't fully developed enough to ward off any potential contaminants that may be found in the honey.

When purchasing honey, choose raw whenever possible. Most commercial honey has been heat-treated and/or pasteurized which destroys the beneficial enzymes found in the honey. Since honey naturally doesn't spoil, it is fundamentally unnecessary to pasteurize it. If you are wanting to take advantage of honey's medicinal qualities in helping with allergies, look for honey that was collected from hives in your area. Watch labels carefully as some commercial honey brands mix in other ingredients to increase profits.

On our homestead, we have a couple of bee hives for pollination and honey collection. The bees are truly fascinating to watch, and I am ever humbled and amazed by the bees. For such a small insect, they are industrious, intelligent, and productive with a complex language and an impressive corporate structure. After spending countless hours over the years watching the bees as they work, and relishing in the enjoyment of fresh, raw honey from our hives, I have a deeper appreciation for this powerful superfood God mentions in Scripture. By far it is my favorite of any of the sweeteners available on the market for its flavor, yes, but also its complexity and deep nutritional and medicinal value. When looking for a sweet addition to your diet, consider opting for the one sweetener God specifically mentions as your first choice, too.

Other Healthy Sweeteners

Other than honey, we do have other healthy sweeteners that come from God. Even though they are not individually mentioned in the Bible like honey is, these sweeteners can also offer that sweet enjoyment without jeopardizing your health. The best sweeteners to choose are those that were created by God (not man), and are in their purest form. One of these sweeteners is an herb called stevia.

Stevia comes from the leaves of the *stevia rebaudiana* plant. When dried and ground into a fine powder, stevia is up to 100 times sweeter than sugar, yet does not affect blood sugar levels. For this reason, next to honey, stevia is one of our favorite sweeteners for most recipes where we want some sweet flavor. Because it is so potent, finding the right balance of how much stevia to use can be tricky, as too much can impart a bitter flavor and too little won't offer enough sweetness. Most commercial stevia is refined, so if you choose to use stevia, research your brands to find the ones that most closely stick with God's design.

AND GOD SAID:

Song of Solomon 5: 1

I have come into my garden, my sister, my bride; I have gathered my myrrh with my spice. I have eaten my honeycomb and my honey; I have drunk my wine and my milk. (NIV)

Isaiah 7: 15

He will be eating curds and honey when he knows enough to reject the wrong and choose the right. (NIV)

Other wonderful sweeteners include maple syrup, molasses, sorghum, yacon, and coconut nectar. These sweeteners all come from the sap of natural, God-created plants and are minimally processed before finding their way to your plate. Choose varieties that are unrefined, pure, and organic when possible. Coconut nectar, or coconut sugar as it is sometimes called, comes from the sap of the coconut trees and is collected much like maple sap is collected to make maple syrup. Of the healthier sweeteners, other than stevia and honey, coconut sugar is naturally low on the glycemic index scale, which is a measurement of how the sweetener ranks based on its effect on blood sugar levels. Coconut sugar is a great choice for baking, in my opinion, as it has a wonderful sweet flavor and blends well with the other ingredients in most recipes. Experiment to find your favorites, and remember to always keep the amounts of sweets you consume in balance. God often warns us of gluttony, and of putting the desires of the flesh above the desires of the spirit.

Sweeteners to Avoid:

Not all sweeteners are created equal, and not all sweeteners are good for you. Unfortunately, the top two most widely consumed sweeteners today also happen to be the most toxic to the body: refined white sugar and high fructose corn syrup. These ingredients can be found in an estimated 60% of packaged foods and drinks at the grocery store, including condiments, dressings, meats, and even commercial milk! (*52) Sugars are often added to many "dead" foods to add flavor back into them after the life-force has been processed out. Other sweeteners commonly used are man-made versions that may taste sweet, but as we have seen time and again, man just can't do as good a job as God in creation.

But what makes unhealthy sweeteners so bad for us? The main reason is how our body recognizes and processes that sweetener. Normally, when you consume a carbohydrate like bread, rice, or grain, the body breaks them down into glucose, the basic form of carbs. Glucose is then easily transported throughout the body to be used as fuel or energy. In contrast, unhealthy sweeteners, particularly refined white sugar and high fructose corn syrup tend to be processed in the body as fructose. Before it can be used as fuel or energy it must be converted into glycogen or fat by the liver. Such high concentrations put excess pressure on our liver, thyroid, and adrenals as these organs attempt to regain balance in the body.

But, you may be thinking, what about the fructose in fruit? I'm so glad you asked! Yes, fruits contain fructose but when you consume them in a whole food, living form, you are also getting the fibers and other parts of the fruit which slows down the digestion and absorption of the fructose. This is why most nutrition experts, when talking about juicing, will say to juice your vegetables but blend your fruits. Fruit juices go directly into the bloodstream and are processed quickly in the liver and converted to fats. All too often I consult with people who think they're doing well and making healthier choices by drinking fruit juices, but then don't understand why they still don't seem to be losing weight. By all means, enjoy your fruit! Just keep the pulp, so your body can properly convert that wonderful goodness into healthy energy!

Unfortunately, many popular fruit juices on the market don't even contain that much fruit. Upon closer inspection of the label, we see the familiar sugar and high fructose corn syrup, among many other unhealthy sweeteners. Let's look closer at the top unhealthy options and the science behind what makes them so detrimental to our health.

Refined White Sugar

Refined white sugar comes from sugarcane, a perennial tropical grass that grows into tall stalks. The stalks are cut, then crushed to extract the juice from the fibers. The juice is then heated and spun to remove all the moisture, leaving sugar crystals. At this point you have raw sugar, which is also sometimes called evaporated cane juice. Raw sugar and evaporated cane juice will have a light tan to dark brown color, since it is still in its natural, unprocessed state.

For some purposes and some recipes, this version isn't too bad as far as healthy sweeteners go, since it is still in a form that contains 'light energy' and minerals, and is closer to what God created. It does have a *much* higher glycemix index level than many other natural sweeteners, so use with caution if you have a health condition that requires attention to blood sugar levels. I do use evaporated cane juice as an ingredient when making kombucha (fermented sweet tea), breads, and certain recipes that need actual sugar rather than honey, coconut sugar, molasses, maple syrup, or stevia.

Refined white sugar is taken through additional processing to get that pure, white, uniform consistency. Raw sugar is washed, bleached, decolorized, recrystalized, dried, and then run through a variety of screens to remove all the minerals and possible impurities in the sugar crystals.

AND GOD SAID:

Ezekiel 16: 13

So you were adorned with gold and silver; your clothes were of fine linen and costly fabrick and embroidered cloth. Your food was honey, olive oil, and the finest flour. You became very beautiful and rose to be royalty. (NIV)

Mark 1: 6

John was clothed with camel's hair and wore a leather belt around his waist, and his diet was locusts and wild honey. (NIV)

The average American adult consumes between 150 and 170 pounds of refined sugars each year, according to a 2017 study by the United States Department of Agriculture (USDA)! (*53) That breaks down to the equivalent of approximately ½ pound of sugar consumed each day! That may seem like an extreme number and not possible, but it's actually easier than you might think. Consider that the average can of soda contains about 8 teaspoons of sugar. Consuming just four 12-ounce cans of soda in a day equates to ¼ pound of sugar! And that's just from soft drinks. Add that to the donuts, cookies, candy, and sugar hidden in processed foods and you easily top ½ pound of sugar each day!

Consuming that much sugar wouldn't be so bad if it weren't so toxic to the body. Refined white sugar contains no nutritional value, is quickly converted into fat in the body, can create imbalances of certain minerals, decreases the immune system's response, and the consumption of refined white sugar has been shown to have negative effects on the body, such as:

- Tooth decay and gum disease
- Obesity
- Migraines
- Imbalanced blood sugar levels
- Allergies
- Arthritis
- Depression
- Behavioral problems
- Insomnia
- Degenerative diseases
- Insulin resistance and diabetes
- Cancer
- High Cholesterol and heart disease

With so many possible side effects to consuming refined white sugar, and with such a high average rate of consumption, it is no wonder that in America we are seeing continued epidemic proportions of health issues such as obesity, diabetes, depression, and cancer. And, to top it off, refined white sugar has been proven to be highly addictive. Cassie Bjork, R.D., L.D., states in a recent study, "Research shows that sugar can be even more addicting than cocaine. Sugar activates the opiate receptors in our brain and affects the reward center, which leads to compulsive behavior, despite the negative consequences like weight gain, headaches, hormone imbalances, and more. Studies suggest that every time we eat [processed sugars] we are reinforcing those neuropathways, causing the brain to become increasingly hardwired to crave sugar, building up a tolerance like any other drug." (*54)

Sugar addiction is a real problem; one to which I can closely relate. For the longest time, I didn't even realize I had such a bad addiction. But working in the corporate world where donuts and chocolate were an almost daily occurrence, and soft drinks were a way of getting through the day, I found myself in a situation that was quickly spiraling out of control. When I learned about sugar addiction, I tried to deny to myself that I had a problem. But when I KNEW I shouldn't eat those things...yet still couldn't seem to stop myself, I couldn't fool myself any longer. Breaking the sugar habit IS possible, and if I did it, then I know you can too! The best way to break the sugar addiction is to first turn to God. After having attempted the cold-turkey-eliminate-all-sweets method, I recommend a more effective approach that you are more likely to stick with long-term: replace refined white sugar foods in your diet with sweets that are God's design. Choose pure, raw honey, stevia, pure maple syrup, or other natural sweetener choices. Grab fruit as your dessert or snack instead of that donut or candy bar. Over time, you will find your body adjusting and your tastes changing. And it gets easier and easier the longer you stick with it!

Note: If you are suffering from a more serious health concern like cancer or diabetes, you may also be dealing with a candida overgrowth. Candida is a harmful pathogen that starts out as a yeast in your digestive system and is generally harmless. However, with the use of pharmaceutical drugs like antibiotics, birth control, and some others, times of serious stress, exposure to certain chemicals, and regular consumption of high levels of sugary foods, can cause the candida to replicate, mutate into bacterial, fungal, or parasitic forms, and become systemic. Some recent clinical studies have linked candida overgrowth as the most common underlying cause of cancer. And the worst part is that sugar feeds the candida. If this is the case for you, it is recommended you contact a healthcare professional familiar with candida and to use more drastic measures to eliminate all sugars, including the aforementioned healthy sweets, for a period of time until the candida has been eradicated. For more information about candida and how it relates to health, visit **www.DitchCandida.com**.

AND GOD SAID:

Psalm 119: 103

How sweet are your words to my taste, sweeter than honey to my mounth! (NIV)

Proverbs 25: 27

Too much honey is bad for you, and so is trying to win too much praise. (GNT)

High Fructose Corn Syrup

Just behind refined white sugar in our list of toxic (yet all too often consumed) sweeteners is high fructose corn syrup (HFCS). To make HFCS, caustic soda is used to remove the kernels from the starch in genetically modified corn. Then, genetically modified enzymes are added to the corn starch with processing to convert some of its glucose into fructose, making it super sweet.

Made popular in the 1970's as a sweetener, particularly in the beverage industry, HFCS was found to be a more cost effective sweetener ingredient, have improved heat stability and functionality, and easy to use yet containing a similar flavor response as regular sucrose. These benefits vastly appealed to commercial food manufactures, and it quickly became adopted as a primary sweetener of choice.

Similar to refined white sugar in its effects on the body, high fructose corn syrup taxes the body in many ways. Containing no nutrient value yet high in calories, there is little or no benefits to the body from its consumption yet being even higher in fructose content than sugar at upwards of 65-90%, high fructose corn syrup tops our list in sweeteners to avoid. A few of the most dangerous effects of regularly consuming HFCS includes:
- Obesity
- Fatty Liver, Liver Disease, and Liver Stress
- High Cholesterol
- High Blood Pressure
- Heart Disease
- Leaky Gut Syndrome
- Diabetes
- Cancer

Interestingly, you won't find high fructose corn syrup at your local grocery store, other than as an ingredient in hundreds of products. This sweetener is only available to retail producers and is not sold as an end product. If it were a healthy option, why is it not available to us like honey or molasses?

Agave

Health food trends, through effective marketing, recently attempted to push agave nectar, or agave syrup, to the forefront of healthy sweetener choices; however, this sweetener is on our list of options to avoid. Although it does originally come from the sap of the agave plant, by the time agave syrup reaches your table, it has been highly processed. Plus, more importantly, the syrup contains very high levels of fructose, which as we've already identified, converts too quickly to fat in the system and taxes the liver, thyroid, and adrenals. For this reason, I don't recommend agave as a healthy sweetener option.

Other Man-Made Sweeteners

Throughout the years, I've seen numerous made-made sweeteners hit the market. Many of these sweeteners are still popular and are often found at restaurants in those yellow, pink, and blue packets. Despite what their marketing efforts would lead us to believe, although they may taste sweet, may have fewer calories, may be economical, and may offer convenience, how can anything produced in a lab be as good or better than what was given us by our Divine Creator? Artificial sweeteners are made in a lab not by God, and therefore also not recommended. Over the years, we have seen a myriad of conflicting reports on the health and safety in consuming these artificial sweeteners, including cancer risks, obesity, and sweet addiction equaling or exceeding refined sugar. Often, these artificial sweeteners contain other chemical components that trigger our cravings, making us want more.

For example, I still remember the first time I tried a popular diet cola soft drink, sweetened with aspartame. It tasted horrible, and I remember thinking that all I could taste were chemicals. But, I was thirsty and that's all that was available at the time, so I took another sip... and another... and another. By about the fourth or fifth sip, I found myself actually enjoying it and wanting more. I didn't like it, and my body was rejecting it, but very quickly transitioned to craving it. How can that be natural?

After getting over my sugar addiction and changing my lifestyle to healthier food choices, I still find myself often amazed when I take a sip or try a bite of something I used to eat regularly and how much different it tastes, and I don't mean in a good way! How quickly our body will adapt to and sometimes even crave things that are so unhealthy. As a general rule, try avoiding foods that were made in a lab rather than those created by God, because no matter how hard and how often we try, man just can't surpass God when it comes to creation. Sweets are no exception. How can something created in a lab contain any "life energy"?

AND GOD SAID:

Judges 14: 18

And the men of the city said unto him on the seventh day before the sun went down, What is sweeter than honey? And what is stronger than a lion? (KJV)

Proverbs 2: 10

When wisdom enters into thine heart and knoledge is sweet unto thy soul, discretion shall preserve thee, understanding shall keep thee. (KJV)

The Many Forms of Unhealthy Sweeteners

When reading ingredients labels, be aware that unhealthy sugar can take many forms. A few ingredients to watch out for and avoid include: acesulfame potassium, advantame, agave, alitame, aspartame, barley malt, beet sugar, brown sugar, buttered sugar, cane juice, caramel color, corn syrup, corn syrup solids, confectioner's sugar, carob syrup, castor sugar, cyclamate, demerara sugar, dextran dextrose, diastatic malt, diatase, ethyl maltol, fructose, fruit juice concentrate, galactose, glucose, glucose solids, golden sugar, golden syrup, high fructose corn syrup, icing sugar, invert sugar, lactose, maltodextrin, maltose, malt syrup, neohesperidine dihydrochalcone, panocha, rice syrup, saccharin, sorbitol, sucralose, sucrose, and tapioca syrup.

Spiritual Significance of Honey and Sweets

Before doing research to write this book, I never really thought much about honey or sweets in the Bible as having any specific spiritual significance. Articles online alluded to honey prophetically referring to the word of God itself, spiritual awakening, deliverance, healing, advancement, making good choices, anointing, and our salvation. After deep reflection and prayer, it became apparent that these interpretations of the spiritual significance of honey seemed to follow a theme; one which follows the general logic of what one might anticipate the meaning of honey to represent.

What comes to mind for you when you think of the word "honey" or the word "sweet"? Deep down in our souls, they represent all things good in our lives.... Like happiness, love, peace, prosperity, salvation, health, cute cuddly baby puppies....you get the idea.

We even often use "honey" as a term of endearment to someone we deeply care about. In your spiritual walk, consider all those things that are good, that are sweet, in your life and let your heart fill with gratitude for God's abundant blessings. No matter how dire the circumstances, no matter how down and out you may feel, no matter how much pain you may be experiencing, God's deep and abounding love is always there. And His blessings can always be found in countless ways.

As we've discussed, sugar is addictive. Granted, there is a physical component to sugar addiction, yet I encourage you to consider the spiritual component as well. Could it be that we may be craving the physical endorphins released when we consume sugar partly because we feel disconnected from God and fill that void in other ways? Could we be turning to 'comfort foods' in an attempt to feel better, only to still feel empty inside... when only God can truly ease that hunger, nourish the spirit, and give you the peace you seek?

AND GOD SAID:

1 Samuel 14: 25

The entire army entered the woods, and there was honey on the ground.

Theologenic Diet
List of Sweets

The following is a summary of sweeteners you can enjoy as discussed in this chapter. Look for options that have been minimally processed and in their purest form. Read labels carefully as not all versions are created equal and ingredients like high fructose corn syrup may be included. It is wise to use all sweets sparingly, particularly those with higher glycemic indexes, and monitor your body's reaction closely.

**Avoid all listed sweeteners other than maybe stevia if you have a candida overgrowth, and see your healthcare provider for recommendations if you have blood sugar issues or diabetes.

Applesauce (organic, unsweetened)
Balsamic Glaze
Banana Puree
Brown Rice Syrup (use sparingly, great corn syrup substitute)
Coconut Nectar, Coconut Sugar
Fruit Puree or Real Fruit Jams (unsweetened)
Dates
Honey
Luo Han Guo (Monk Fruit)
Maple Syrup
Molasses
Raw Cane Sugar (use sparingly)
Sorghum
Stevia
Yacon Syrup

Tips:
- Chocolate is a favorite sweet treat for many. If you are making chocolate desserts, try using cacao powder instead of cocoa powder. Cacao powder is the unprocessed and raw form of chocolate, contains valuable minerals like magnesium, and is considered a superfood.
- Commercial chocolate bars or chocolate chips can now be found sweetened with stevia rather than sugar. Try these versions, like Lily's Brand, for your chocolate recipes.
- Unsweetened applesauce or banana puree make great sweetener substitutes in many recipes.
- Dates are a wonderful way to sweeten recipes without using sugar, and are mentioned specifically in the Bible. Check out our Recipe section for "Date Honey" which can be used in recipes or as a spread.

Chapter Summary:

Although sweets are a popular favorite in our diets, not all sweets are created equal and most are quite hazardous to our health. The only true sweetener found in the Bible is honey, and even then God specifically tells us to exercise moderation. Other acceptable sweeteners are those that are created by God and in their purest form. Processed and refined sweeteners and man-made sweeteners are not recommended, as they have been proven through countless studies and scientific evidence to be toxic, cause numerous health issues, and be addictive. We can still enjoy the pleasure of sweet treats from time to time, in the form of wholesome ingredients that have "life energy."

Action Steps:

1. Take a personal assessment of how much sugar you are currently consuming on a daily basis, taking into account the sugar found in processed foods, boxed foods, jarred foods, packaged foods, beverages, and even meats. Make the commitment to avoid foods containing unhealthy sweeteners.
2. Do you have a sugar addiction? Recognition is the first step. Then, work with God to make better choices, reducing your sugar consumption and replacing all unhealthy sweets with healthy sweets. If you are faced with a major health concern, consider eliminating all sweets for a period of at least 21 days, using only stevia or monk fruit to satisfy your sweet cravings to allow your body to recover and heal.
3. Switch to fresh fruit, whenever possible, as a dessert or sweet snack.
4. Take a moment each day to thank and praise God for all the abundant blessings you have in your life; for all those wonderful sweet gifts. Seek to live a life with a heart filled with gratitude and love.

Notes:

Chapter 10: Olive Oil, Oils, & Fats

Physical Significance of Olive Oil, Oils, & Fats

Generally speaking, when talking about nutrition, most dieticians will focus on the big three: Proteins, Carbohydrates, and Fats. Over the years, public opinion on consuming fats has changed from loving them, to hating them, to loving them again. Once again, colorful and convincing marketing campaigns have used creative techniques to convince us that "low fat" is the way to go if you want to lose weight and get healthy. Or, conversely, new fad diets extol the benefits of consuming lots of fat, with the claims that high fat foods help reset the metabolism and you will lose weight. Unfortunately, both "low fat" and "high fat" trends are examples of misguided attempts which have mis-led countless individuals into unhealthy situations and bad habits.

The truth is that fats are a crucial part of health, as long as you consume the right kinds of fats and in the right balance according to how much your body needs for your activity level. Our bodies need fat for energy (about 25% of our energy requirements comes from fat sources), absorption of certain nutrients (fats help us absorb fat-soluble vitamins like A, D, E, and K), and for maintaining our core body temperature.

Not all fats are created equal, however. Typically, dieticians will divide fats into four main categories: Monounsaturated Fats, Polyunsaturated Fats, Saturated Fats, and Trans Fats. Classification into these categories is determined by the chemical structure of the fat itself.

- Monounsaturated Fats have a chemical structure where the fat molecules have one unsaturated carbon bond in the molecule, also called a double bond, with the remainder single-bond. These fats are liquid at room temperature, but can start to turn solid when chilled.
- Polyunsaturated Fats are similar but have more than one double bond, and are generally liquid at both room temperature and when chilled.
- Saturated Fats do not have double bonds and are solids at room temperature or chilled, and can become liquid when heated.
- Trans Fats, or trans fatty acids, are fats that have been created in an industrial process that adds hydrogen to liquid oils to make them more solid.

AND GOD SAID:

Leviticus 24: 2

Command the sons of Israel that they bring you clear oil from beaten olives for the light, to make a lamp burn continually.

Exodus 29: 40

And there shall be one-tenth of an ephah of fine flour mixed with one-fourth of a hin of olive oil, and one forth of a hin of whine for a drink offering with one lamb.

I remember learning about the various types of fats back in middle school health class. Back then, these terms all seemed to blend together and when the teacher was talking about them, I found my eyes somewhat glazing over. All these scientific terms with complex names and meanings seemed so confusing. What does all this really mean, and what do I really need to know so I can make better decisions for my health? If you feel like I did, before you tune out and before your eyes, too, start glazing over, let's break it down into simple terms along with what scripture says about which are the best fats to choose.

The Best Fats for Health

The best sources for fat in our diet, particularly if you aren't cooking them, are those that are monounsaturated or polyunsaturated fats in the form of oils. Examples of healthy oils include extra virgin olive oil, sunflower oil, avocado oil, sesame oil, almond oil, and pumpkin seed oil for monounsaturated, and flaxseed oil, walnut oil, fish oils, safflower oil, and hemp seed oil for polyunsaturated.

In the Bible, the most common word for oil is the Hebrew word *shemen*, which largely refers to olive oil and is found approximately 190 times. Olive oil was a highly valued commodity and was used with food, ceremonies, anointing and worship, and as a fuel for their lamps. No other oil is mentioned as often as olive oil and scientific studies further support that olive oil is one of the best choices we can make when our goal is adding healthy fat to our diet. Olive oil is a monounsaturated fat, contains large amounts of antioxidants, is loaded with nutrients, has strong anti-inflammatory properties, and tastes amazing. What's not to love about that?

Scientifically, monounsaturated fats like olive oil have been proven to reduce bad cholesterol levels in the blood, lower the risk of heart disease, lower the risk of stroke, improve insulin sensitivity, support liver health, help balance hormones, fight depression, and encourage weight loss.

One important consideration when looking at monounsaturated or polyunsaturated fats, however, is that since they contain double bonds, they are more volatile when heated. Heating healthy oils above a certain temperature (which varies for each oil, and is lower than most cooking temperatures) can cause heat-induced damage, change the molecular structure, and potentially decrease the health benefits. Therefore, for cooking purposes, we turn to a different type of fat.

Fats that are Good for Health when used in Moderation

Saturated fats, or those that are solid at room temperature, generally get a lot of negative press when it comes to health. These fats, like butter, ghee, coconut oil, and palm kernel oil, have been falsely accused of causing health problems. This misunderstanding came from a series of studies done in the early part of the 20th century when heart disease started becoming a bigger problem. In these studies, it was found that high cholesterol could be linked to heart disease. They also found in other studies that some saturated fats (not all) could raise cholesterol levels. The assumption was then made that saturated fats could be therefore linked to heart disease. Even though this assumption has since been clinically proven in countless studies to be incorrect, the stigma has carried on. (*56)

In reality, saturated fats, assuming you are choosing those that were derived from organic and/or grass-fed sources, make an excellent fat choice when cooking. Because they have no double bonds, saturated fats are very stable when heated. Plus, they add wonderful flavor to the foods in which they are cooked.

Health benefits of saturated fats, when consumed in moderation, include stronger bones, improved liver health, healthy lungs, proper nerve signaling, a stronger immune system, and a healthy brain. (*57)

When choosing saturated fats for cooking, stick with those that come from sources approved by scripture (meaning they come from God, relatively pure, and not made from pork fat).

Coconut Oil

For example, coconut oil is an excellent choice. Although coconuts are not specifically mentioned in scripture, they grow on palm trees, which *are* mentioned is several verses. Coconut oil is made from the white flesh inside the coconut fruit. The best coconut oils are those that are virgin, expeller pressed, wet milled, or unrefined organic coconut oil as these versions will still have the most "life energy" in them. Refined versions tend to have been heated or processed, which reduces the health benefits of the oil. Coconut oil has been found in over 1500

AND GOD SAID:

Psalm 92:12

The righteous shall flourish like the palm tree; he shall grow like a cedar in Lebanon.

Isaiah 7: 15

Butter and honey shall he eat, that he may know to refule the evil, and choose the good. (KJV)

studies to be a healthy choice, particularly because coconut oil is comprised of medium-chain fatty acids like caprylic acid, lauric acid, and capric acid. This means that coconut oil is easier on the digestive system, is processed by the liver which means it is immediately converted into energy and not stored as fat by the body, and contains anti microbial and anti fungal properties. (*58) My husband makes the best popcorn, and he says one of his secrets is that he pops it the old fashioned way (on the stove...no microwave version here) with coconut oil. So yummy!

Butter

Another excellent choice is good ol' fashioned butter. Butter is made from dairy, so the best butter is made from grass-fed, organic, A2 beta-casein milk. Now, before you shake your head and discount butter as a healthy choice, consider whether your opinions about butter are based on science and biblical principles. For years, butter has been getting bad publicity, fueled in part by the margarine industry. But the reality is that butter has many health benefits, tastes great, and is mentioned in the Bible several times. Most of the bad publicity revolved around butter as a cause for heart disease and high cholesterol. Scientists now know, however, that cholesterol comes in two forms, HDL (high density lipoprotein) and LDL (low density lipoprotein). HDL cholesterol is beneficial to the body, particularly during times of stress or when injury or inflammation is present. Interestingly, low blood cholesterol levels have been associated with side-effects such as a higher risk of depression, a higher risk of violent crimes or suicide, and a higher risk of dementia! (*59)

LDL cholesterol, generally thought of as "bad cholesterol", can be subcategorized into large, fluffy LDL particles and small, dense LDL particles. Only the small, dense LDL particles are harmful to the body. Saturated fats like butter and coconut oil can actually change the dense LDL particles back to the fluffy LDL particles. I know I'm getting a little technical again, but in order to fully understand the difference and possibly break some old paradigms you may be carrying, we needed to get a bit specific. Primary sources of LDL cholesterol are found in highly processed oils and processed meats. If you are concerned with cholesterol, it is important that you fully understand the difference and how choosing fats with "life energy," instead of process or "dead energy" fats ,can actually help.

And that's not all! Butter contains conjugated linoleic acid and butyric acid, fatty acids that both have been proven to inhibit the growth of cancer! Butter also is loaded with fat soluble vitamins like K2!

Here on our homestead, we enjoy occasionally making butter from scratch. It's a fun project to do with the kids, and there's nothing like fresh butter on some fresh baked bread! We simply take cream and whip it until the butter fat separates from the buttermilk. We then strain off the buttermilk (we use this to make the best pancakes ever!), add a little salt (and maybe some honey), and enjoy!

Ghee

A lesser known healthy saturated fat is ghee. Ghee, sometimes called clarified butter, is made by heating butter slowly to separate the butterfat from the milk solids, which are then skimmed off. With the milk solids removed, you are left with just the butterfat. As a result, you are left with a delicious, creamy substance that:

- has little casein or lactose (most are removed with the milk solids) making ghee a great choice even for those with dairy sensitivities.
- has a higher smoke point (temperature at which the fat begins to oxidize) at 485°F making it an excellent choice for higher heat cooking like pan-frying or baking.
- blends well with spices, and often enhances their flavors.

Whether you choose butter, ghee, or both, choose grass-fed, organic whenever possible for maximum health benefits and nutrients. Either way, I encourage you to give them a try and experience the delicious difference for yourself.

Unhealthy Fats You Should Avoid

Unfortunately, the unhealthy fats are what gives the healthy fats a bad reputation (guilty by association), and there are many of them. At the top of our list for unhealthy fats to avoid are the highly processed or Trans Fats. Common Trans Fats include margarine, hydrogenated oils, and partially hydrogenated oils. These fats have generally been derived by adding hydrogen to liquid vegetable oils to make them more solid. Essentially, the molecular structure of the oil has been changed. The results may be more shelf-stable, inexpensive, and hold up for longer periods of high heat (popular for deep-fat frying), but these benefits are

AND GOD SAID:

Leviticus 2: 6

Crumble it into morsels of bread and then pour olive oil on it.

2 Chronicles 2: 15

Now let my lord send to his servants the wheat, barley, olive oil, and wine he has promised.

only good for big businesses, not you, the consumer. Trans Fats are high in the bad, dense, LDL cholesterol which increases the risk of heart disease, heart attacks, and stroke. Trans Fats also contribute to weight gain and obesity.

A common Trans Fat to avoid is Crisco. I remember one time when I was a kid and my mom left the container of Crisco out in the barn. I was young enough that I don't remember *why* it got left out there, but I do remember that after a couple months, that container looked *exactly* the same! No bugs, no flies, no decay, no mold, no melting, nothing! Even as a kid, I could recognize that there was something wrong about that! If the bugs don't even want to eat it, then why would we?

Another common Trans Fat is hydrogenated (and partially hydrogenated) oil. These oils are often found in processed foods because they add flavor and extend the shelf life. However, hydrogenated and partially hydrogenated oils have been proven to cause serious damage to the body, even in small amounts, including inflammation, hardening of the arteries, hormone disruption, block certain chemical receptors, and contribute to numerous chronic diseases such as heart disease, stroke, diabetes, and cancer. As much as we may love those fast food, fried, or processed choices, they just don't follow God's plan of "life energy" and health.

You may be surprised by the next oils we list as unhealthy and to avoid, but I highly recommend you take them off your list of pantry items. These are common oils and some of the most widely consumed in the United States, and include vegetable oil, soybean oil, corn oil, peanut oil, and canola oil. Canola oil? Yep, you read that correctly. Even though canola oil is a polyunsaturated fat and has been touted to be a "healthy" oil, along with all the other oils listed, it is a highly processed oil that is unhealthy. Canola oil, by the time you consume it, has been refined, bleached, deodorized, and heated; unless you find unrefined, virgin canola oil (which is very hard to find and quite expensive). Generally with all oils, the more they are processed, the less health benefits they offer. With so many other healthier oil and fat choices out there, why take the risk on a processed oil that could not only be unhealthy, but potentially life threatening?

The last unhealthy fat that bears mentioning is lard. My grandma cooked with lard and insisted that the secret to the best chocolate chip cookies was to use lard instead of butter. However, lard is made from pig fat, which as we have already discussed is definitely not God's design for health. Lard also is much higher in saturated fats, including the "bad" LDL cholesterol. As good as those cookies may be, they're just not worth the risks.

Spiritual Significance of Olive Oil

Olive oil was a highly valued commodity during Biblical times. The first mention of oil extraction took place during the Exodus from Egypt, where the oil was derived by hand squeezing and stored in special containers under the watchful guard of the priests. This oil was also sometimes referred to as "sweet oil" as it was quite fragrant. Conversely, olive oil was also derived mechanically, by crushing, stamping, and squeezing the olives with stones. This oil, although still valuable, was not acceptable as an anointing oil and did not have the fragrance or flavor as the sweet oil. Spiritually, when we accept Christ into our hearts, will be as the sweet oil and be a fragrant offering to the Lord, or will we be hard-pressed and remain tasteless to the world?

Olives are a bitter fruit, and to make them into a sweet, aromatic, and flavorful oil, these bitter globes are squeezed under extreme pressure. During this process of strife, the sweet oil emerges. What pressures are you facing now, that God is using to extract something better from you?

AND GOD SAID:

2 Corinthians 2: 15

For we are to God the pleasing aroma of Christ among those who are being saved and those who are perishing. (NIV)

Theologenic Diet
List of Oils and Fats

The following is a summary of oils and fats you can enjoy as discussed in this chapter. Look for options that have been minimally processed and in their purest form, such as extra virgin, expeller pressed, or raw. Animal fats should be grass-fed and organic. Read labels carefully to avoid any unhealthy fats.

Best Oils for High Temperature or Cooking:

Coconut Oil
Butter
Ghee
Palm Kernel Oil (non-processed)

Best Oils for Low Temperature Preparations (Virgin, Expeller Pressed, or Raw)

Olive Oil
Avocado Oil
Sesame Oil
Pumpkin Seed Oil
Hempseed Oil
Sunflower Oil
Cod Liver Oil
Flaxseed Oil
Almond Oil
Walnut Oil
Safflower Oil
Grapeseed Oil

Excellent Food Sources for Healthy Fats

Nuts, Nut Milks, and Nut Butters
Seeds like chia, flax, sesame, sunflower
Avocado
Olives
Tahini
Eggs
Whole Milk
Fish
Grass-Fed, Organic Meats on God's Allowed List
Dark Chocolate

Oils and Fats to Avoid

Partially hydrogenated oils
Hydrogenated oils
Margarine
Lard
Canola oil
Peanut oil
Vegetable oil
Corn oil
Soybean oil

Note: Most restaurants use one or more of these oils when preparing foods, particularly deep fat fried foods.

Chapter Summary:

Fats are an important part of any healthy diet, particularly because they offer such a great source of energy, however not all fats are created equal. Scripture specifically mentions Olive Oil as a wonderful source of fat for cooking, medicinal purposes, and ceremony. Other healthy fats are those that contain the most "life energy" and have not been heavily processed. Animal fat sources such as those found in butter, cheese, and ghee, especially when they come from grass-fed, organically raised A2 beta-casein milk are excellent healthy choices when consumed in moderation.

Action Steps:

1. If you haven't already, eliminate processed and "dead" foods from your diet. These foods contain unhealthy trans fats that, along with many other harmful ingredients, are adding to your health risks.
2. Assess which fats and oils you are currently consuming regularly. Make adjustments as needed to healthier options both for high heat and low heat preparations.
3. Some healthy fats are needed every day for optimum health, but too much of a good thing can become a bad thing. Fats, even healthy fats, are higher in calories and therefore give you more energy. But, you'll want to consume the right amount for your activity level.
4. Prayerfully consider what areas of your life you are being "squeezed" right now, in order for God to work with you to extract your sweet oil. How will you then use that sweet oil to better fuel your lamp to let your inner light shine?

Notes:

Chapter 11: Wine, Vinegar, & Other Beverages

Physical Significance of Wine, Vinegar, & Other Beverages

Staying hydrated is a crucial cornerstone to health by drinking enough fresh water. Sometimes, however, we want to enjoy other beverages for variety and flavor. Some options are better than others, and not all beverages are going to support health or follow God's plan. Let's take a quick look at a few popular choices and what God and science say about them for health.

Wine

When I was in college, I had the amazing opportunity to study abroad in France for a semester. Spending time internationally really opened my eyes at a young age to the diversity of this world and how deeply our culture and history play a role in our lives. While in France, my host family introduced me to the traditions and complexities of wine and wine making. Although at first I didn't really care for the taste, I came to truly appreciate the deep history surrounding this fermented beverage.

One of the most well known "foods" mentioned in the Bible is wine. Turning water into wine was Jesus' first miracle, wine was included in the Last Supper, and wine often graced the celebration tables of scripture. God's guidelines about wine and other alcoholic beverages is a controversial subject, however. On one side are those who advocate drinking wine as long as it is in moderation, proven by scriptural verses. On the other side are those who say complete abstinence and avoidance of any and all alcohol are required, since scripture warns against alcohol and it is historically unclear whether the wine of the Bible contained alcohol at all. It is not the goal of this book to change your mind, depending on which side you may fall. If you don't consume any alcohol, by all means please continue. If your interpretation allows for the occasional consumption (emphasis on occasional), it is important that you understand a few things science has proven about wine. It is also important to keep in mind that while scripture often mentions wine, there are also many scriptures about not consuming too much, avoiding drunkenness, and avoiding gluttony.

AND GOD SAID:

Mark 14: 23-24

And when He had taken a cup and given thanks, He gave it to them, and they all drank from it. And He said to them, "This is My blood of the covenant, which is poured out for many.

Isaiah 25:6

The LORD of hosts will prepare a lavish banquet for all peoples on this mountain; A banquet of aged wine, choice pieces with marrow, And refined, aged wine.

With wine, it is also important to understand that although wine can offer some health benefits such as supporting the heart and circulatory system through the polyphenols and antioxidants found in red wine in particular, the wine of Bible times was much different than the wine typically consumed today. Wine is made from grapes, and grape varieties, growing methods, and use of pesticides has changed over the years, along with the processing techniques and preparation methods. Modern wine is much stronger, with a higher alcohol content, a higher sugar content, and higher traces of residual toxins than the wine of the Bible. For these reasons, it is highly recommended to avoid consuming wine, even if in moderation. Science proves that any and all alcohol kills brains cells (which you can never get back), contributes to dehydration, has an acidifying effect on the body, and feeds harmful yeasts and fungus in the body.

Regular excessive consumption of alcohol can also create an addiction. If you currently find yourself in a situation where you have an addiction to alcohol (or anything else), I highly advise you to seek professional help. God has bigger plans for your life, and some challenges are better faced with support.

Vinegar

In the process of making wine, the grapes go through several stages of fermentation. At times, the fermentation can continue to the point where natural bacteria in the brew consume the alcohol and turn it into vinegar. Some interpretations of certain scriptural verses portray the use of vinegar rather than wine. Vinegar is a wonderful healthy addition to the diet. Scientifically, vinegar has been shown to be beneficial to the body, particularly for the digestive system and immune system.

One study, published in 2016 showed that consuming 2 tablespoons of apple cider vinegar before bedtime with a healthy snack balanced blood sugar levels on test subjects with Type 2 Diabetes. (*60) Other studies have shown apple cider vinegar to help with digestive health, aide in weight loss, reduce bad cholesterol levels, and support the immune system.

Vinegar, contains acetic acid, which, like other acidic foods we consume, like lemon juice, increases the absorption of valuable minerals in the digestive process, particularly calcium. Dairy products and dark, leafy greens are excellent sources of calcium, yet adding a splash of vinegar to those greens can greatly increase the body's ability to utilize the calcium in those foods.

The acetic acid in vinegar also slows down the conversion of carbohydrates into sugars in the bloodstream. This is especially valuable to diabetics and can reduce spikes of blood sugar levels, allowing the body's natural regulation response to keep things in balance.

Additionally, vinegar helps support the beneficial bacteria in the digestive system. Science is starting to realize the importance and impact of the good bacteria found in our bodies. The average adult has upwards of 10 trillion bacteria in the body, aiding with key functions such as brain function, hormones, moods, digestion, nutrient absorption, and immune system. A balanced and healthy good bacterial flora, particularly in the digestive system, is cornerstone to health. *The more we can support our good bacteria, the better our health and ability to stay healthy.* Vinegars are one way of supporting the good bacteria.

Kombucha

Another way to support the good bacteria is by drinking kombucha. Kombucha is one of my favorite beverages and is an excellent soft drink replacement since it has a nice "fizz". If you're not familiar with kombucha, it is probiotic tea, a living food, composed of tea, good bacteria strains, and good yeast strains. I was first introduced to kombucha by my sister-in-law, who gave me my first "starter" and taught me how to make it. From the first time I tried this flavorful beverage, I was hooked. Delicious, easy to make, and loaded with benefits to the body, kombucha quickly became a staple item in our refrigerator and regularly graces our table.

Kombucha has been shown to be particularly beneficial to the liver and kidneys, supports the digestive process, supports healthy elimination of waste, supports the immune system, reduces inflammation in the body, and helps the body with detoxifying and eliminating heavy metal build up in the system. Kombucha is such a powerful detoxifier, it has been used successfully during cancer treatment, supporting the body during and after treatment, and supporting the body's recovery after exposure to radiation and heavy toxins.

Some biblical scholars believe that it was kombucha that was served to Ruth as found in Ruth 2:14. In this verse we read about how the land-owner Boas invited the Moabite Ruth, who later became his wife, during her gleaning of grains: "Come over here and eat some bread and dip your morsel into the vinegar-drink! And she sat down beside the reapers; and he reached her parched corn and she ate and

AND GOD SAID:

John 19:28-29

After this, Jesus, knowing that all things had already been accomplished, to fulfill the Scripture, said, "I am thirsty." A jar full of sour wine was standing there; so they put a sponge full of the sour wine upon a branch of hyssop and brought it up to His mouth.

Ruth 2: 14

Come over here and eat some bread and dip your morsel into the vinegar-drink! And she sat down beside the reapers; and he reached her parched corn and she ate and was sufficed and left.

was sufficed and left." This biblical report of a vinegar-drink, kombucha or not, shows how the people during this time saw the value of beverages containing microorganism of lactic acid to provide strength and refreshment during the hard work of the harvest season.

If you've never tried kombucha, I recommend checking it out, especially if you are looking for a healthier alternative to soft drinks and soda. I have found that drinking kombucha also helps with curbing sugar cravings, too! If you can get your hands on a "starter", I encourage you to make it yourself. It's super easy, you get to control the ingredients and the flavor, and making it yourself is extremely economical. My family drinks about two gallons of kombucha each week, and I spend less than 15 minutes making this powerhouse probiotic-rich drink. And the kids absolutely love it!

For your convenience, we offer a full online tutorial on how to make kombucha on our website at www.HealthyHomesteadLiving.com or www.TheLivingFoodsAcademy.com where we walk you through everything you need to know about maximizing the benefits of this awesome superfood beverage.

Kvass

Another living beverage, infused with beneficial good bacteria, is kvass. Kvass is made by infusing either fruits or vegetables with beneficial bacteria and allowing the brew to ferment. A popular kvass is made using beets and onions. Traditional kvass is made using sourdough rye bread and has a deep earthy, salty, and somewhat tangy flavor. Loaded with beneficial bacteria, B vitamins, and manganese, kvass is often used as a digestive tonic, blood tonic, cancer fighter, liver cleanser, and detoxifyer.

Less common than kombucha, kvass is not found commercially as often, but it is very easy to make and doesn't require any special equipment or tools other than a glass jar. The benefits of making it yourself is you can adjust the ingredients according to your personal tastes. In our house, I enjoy beet kvass, but my daughter and husband much prefer peach kvass. Either way, kvass offers another delicious superfood beverage loaded with beneficial bacteria to support the gut and consequently overall health.

Coffee

Coffee has become one of the most widely consumed beverages on the planet, and coffee drinkers have a particular affinity to their brew. My husband used to love his morning coffee and that tantalizing aroma as I prepared it for him did stimulate the senses.

However, when we found out that he had high blood pressure, one of the first things we did was eliminate the coffee. Coffee, when consumed in excess, can have negative health effects including increased blood pressure, increased heart rate, muscle tremors and jitters, heartburn, anxiety, dehydration, insomnia, headaches, and ulcers. In my research on the health effects of drinking coffee, I came across a study done by a Dr. Tainio. He was studying the energy of the body and found that most healthy adults have an energetic frequency of around 62-68 MHz. When a person's frequency lowers to 58 MHz, the risk of getting a cold increases. Flu symptoms start at 57 MHz, candida at 55 MHz, and cancer at 42 MHz. The process of dying begins at 25 MHz and goes to zero at death. Dr. Tainio further found that just holding a cup of coffee could lower the body frequency by 8 MHz and that by taking a sip can lower one's frequency by 14 Mhz! In most test cases, the subject took three days to recover energy frequency lost from just one sip of coffee. (*67)

Coffee also contains caffeine, which is a stimulant and puts stress on the adrenal system and nervous system. Caffeine can be a highly addictive substance, and can be classified as a neurotoxin, meaning that it affects and causes damage to the nervous system and the brain. Eliminating coffee, like any addictive substance or drug, can cause withdrawal symptoms like headaches and lethargy. These side effects only last for a couple of days, though, so stick with it and you'll feel so much better afterwards. Coffee is not mentioned in the Bible, and the negative effects on the body far outweigh any possible benefits.

Tea

After water, tea is the most widely consumed beverage in the world, followed closely by coffee. Tea is made by steeping the cured leaves of the Camellia sinensis plant in hot or boiling water for a period of time. Tea leaves can be found as black, green, oolong, red (rooibos), and white; the only difference being on the process used for curing the leaves. Tea contains antioxidants and has been found to be beneficial to the heart, be hydrating to the body (despite the caffeine), fight depression, and boost the metabolism. One study found green tea to improve bone mineral density. (*61)

AND GOD SAID:

Psalm 69: 21

They gave me also gall for my meat; and in my thirst they gave me vinegar to drink.

153

1 Timothy 5: 23

Stop drinking only water, and use a little vinegar because of your stomach and your frequent illnesses.

A good tea can be mixed with a variety of herbs, fruits, and spices to make some truly delicious concoctions that are satisfying and nutritious. As with any commercially purchased food product, look for organic, free-trade options. I also generally recommend going with loose tea rather than the tea bags. Although the tea bags may be convenient, they often contain the dusty remnants and are much inferior quality. By using loose leaf tea, you can visually see the quality of the tea you are making.

Tea aficionados are quite adamant that there are right ways and wrong ways to brew a good cup of tea. Right way or wrong way, as with anything, moderation and balance are key. Due to the caffeine levels found in tea, avoid overdoing how much you consume. Any consumption of caffeine can have negative effects on the body, particularly the nervous system and the brain. If you have trouble sleeping, you also may want to avoid drinking any beverage containing caffeine after 4 p.m.

Herbal teas, on the other hand, are made from steeping one or a variety of herbs in boiling water to extract the health benefits of the leaves, roots, or stems. Where regular tea should be consumed in moderation due to the caffeine it consumes, herbal teas can be enjoyed regularly. Know your herbs, and be cautious of any reactions with medications you may be taking. Herbs are God's medicines, with a myriad of benefits, however you'll want to contact a professional if you have a specific health concern.

Soft Drinks

Soft drinks, or sodas, should be completely avoided. I know you may give me some resistance on this one, but hear me out. Modern commercial soft drinks have evolved over the years to be full of incredibly toxic substances and chemicals with few ingredients of any nutritional value. Soft drink companies spend vast amounts of money to find the perfect combinations of flavors and sweeteners to tap into the part of your brain that makes you crave more.

The term "soft drink" originated to distinguish flavored drinks from hard liquor or distilled spirits (alcoholic beverages). Early marketing of these flavored beverages, usually made with a combination of fruits, sweeteners, and natural flavors, were to recommend these beverage choices as a substitute to their alcoholic counterparts. These early versions may not have been so bad from a health standpoint, but over the years the soft drink industry has evolved to create what research is now showing, for example, that just two servings a day of soft drinks can significantly increase the risks for metabolic syndrome, type 2 diabetes, heart disease, obesity, and tooth decay.

To give you an idea of how toxic soft drinks can be, let me share a couple personal experiences. My husband has a friend who used to work as an executive for a leading soft drink company. This friend has been retired for his position for years, but he told us once how one of his main jobs when he first started was to find good sources across the globe for the secret spices that went into their signature flavor. By the time he retired, all of those ingredients had been replaced by a chemical synthetic version of the original God-created spice. Not one ingredient was still in its natural form! On another occasion, I was visiting with one of my holistic healthcare friends. He mentioned that one of the worst things about soft drinks is that many of the top brands include bromine or a variation of bromine. Bromine is a highly toxic substance that is actually corrosive to human tissue in a liquid state and causes damage to the liver, kidneys, lungs, stomach, and gastrointestinal tract. He stated that the average can of soda, is so toxic that it paralyzes the immune system for as much as eight hours! And, how often is one can not enough? If you are resistant to giving up your soda, consider the reasoning and whether you are letting earthly reasons stop you from making better choices. Switch to healthier options like kombucha where you can still get fizz and flavor without the harmful effects.

Sports Drinks, Energy Drinks, & Flavored Waters

Other beverages to avoid include sports drinks, energy drinks, and commercially flavored waters. These drinks are often marketed as healthy, however look closely at the ingredients. Do they contain only God created "life energy" ingredients or do they contain unpronounceable or unrecognizable ones? Sports drinks, especially, often contain sugars and unhealthy salts. A better alternative if you need hydration and electrolytes is water with healthy salts like Celtic or Himalayan, lemon, cucumber, and juiced greens. If you need a boost of energy, rather than turn to a chemical beverage that just causes you to crash afterwards, try peppermint essential oil, deep breathing, and energy acupoints such as the outside of the shin, about three fingers down from the knee.

AND GOD SAID:

1 Peter 2: 9

But you are a chosen people, a royal priesthood, a holy nation, God's special possession, that you may declare the praises of him who called you out of darkness into his wonderful light.

Spiritual Significance of Wine & Vinegar

*In the ancient Near East, with its scarcity of water, wine was a necessity rather than a luxury, so it came to symbolize sustenance and life. Due to its close relationship to the ongoing life of the community, in association with grain and oil, wine is also representative of the covenant blessings God promised to Israel for obedience, and which He would withhold for disobedience. Finally, wine also represents joy, celebration, and festivity, expressing the abundant blessings of God. (*62)*

Wine has come to represent many things spiritually, most notably the very blood of Jesus. There is deep symbolism in the wine of the Last Supper. Jesus makes it very clear to His disciples, and to us, that without His paying for the penalty of our sins, we wouldn't have a future other than death. We would have no hope at all. Jesus not only paid the penalty of our sins, He also supplies the spiritual nourishment to produce fruit (represented in the grapes of the wine) that glorifies the Father and prepares us for life in God's Kingdom.

When we partake of the wine during communion, we are reminded of this sacrifice, the hope He offers, and the responsibility we carry to continue as His disciples, fulfilling our destiny through obedience and gratitude.

Theologenic Diet
List of Healthy Beverages

The following is a summary of healthy beverages as outlined in this chapter, along with other beverage suggestions as discussed previously in this book. The vinegars included in this section can be added to beverages or used as condiment ingredients. This list is by no means complete, but will give you a good starting point in making healthier choices.

Water!!!!!
Lemon Water or Fresh, Sugar-free
Lemonade
Coconut Water
Aloe Vera Juice
Apple cider vinegar (with the mother)
White vinegar
Balsamic vinegar
Wine vinegar
Rice vinegar
Malt vinegar
Kombucha
Kefir
Water Kefir
Beet Kvass
Peach Kvass (and other fruit kvass')
Other fruit or vegetable kvass'
Jung (similar to kombucha but made
with
     honey)
Black tea
Green tea
Oolong tea
White tea
Rooibos tea
Matcha tea
Herbal teas (see more in our chapter
on
     herbs)
Green juice (juices from leafy greens
such
     as wheatgrass, kale, spinach,
     etc.)
Fresh vegetable juices
Raw, dark, hot chocolate
A2/A2 organic milk

Drink in Moderation
Coffee (organic, fair-trade, but only
     consumed rarely)
Fresh fruit juices, with the pulp

Beverages to Avoid

Soft Drinks
Sports Drinks
Energy Drinks
Commercial Flavored Waters
Alcoholic Beverages
Fruit Juices from Concentrate

Chapter Summary:

Staying hydrated is important as discussed in our chapter on water, however there are many additional beverage choices that offer health benefits and offer delicious variety and flavors. Other beverages, like soft drinks, should be completely avoided due to the potentially harmful ingredients they contain. Some of the best healthy beverages include those that contain living beneficial bacteria like kombucha, kefir, kvass, and vinegars. Wine and coffee may offer some health benefits, however the risks far outweigh the benefits so consume only occasionally and if your body is healthy enough to handle it.

Action Steps:

1. Make sure you are consuming enough water to stay hydrated (half your body weight in ounces).
2. Start consuming probiotic beverages like kombucha, kefir, or kvass regularly (best if you can add a bit at least once every day, especially if you have health issues).
3. If you consume coffee or wine regularly, assess whether you are getting a balanced and moderate amount that is maximizing the health benefits rather than taxing the body. Consider drastically reducing how much you consume and switch to healthier options.
4. Cut out all soft drinks, sports drinks, energy drinks, or other beverages that contain harmful and toxic ingredients.
5. Attend a church service and partake in Holy Communion, giving thanks for the sacrifice made through the body and blood (bread and wine) for our sins.

Notes:

Chapter 12: Essential Oils & Herbs

Physical Significance of Oils & Herbs

I've always found oils and herbs fascinating. Such amazing gifts God has given us in the form of natural leaves, flowers, roots, bark, and stems from so many plants that carry medicinal and nutritional qualities. I could dedicate a whole book just on each as there are so many varieties of plants, their uses, what they do for the body, and how to best utilize them. Scripturally we find over 1031 verses referencing the use of these powerful and beneficial oils and herbs, with specific reference to 33 species. Used frequently in medicine, worship, cuisine, and ceremony, oils, herbs, and bitters played an important role during biblical times, throughout history, and are slowly making a valiant comeback into our modern health practices. In this chapter, I am going to share with you a few of my favorites, specifically those mentioned in scripture, share a bit about what makes them so powerful, and how to get started using them. I encourage you to experiment, seek out more information, and keep learning about these amazing tools God gives us.

At first, when I was getting started learning about essential oils and herbs, my husband was quite skeptical. Having been raised to stick with traditional medicine for just about anything that ails you, he was hesitant to trust what he called my "concoctions". After experiencing the almost miraculous changes for himself, however, he quickly started changing his tune. My daughter, on the other hand, was pretty much raised with these "alternative" therapies. For her, it is just a natural thing to put onions on the bottom of her feet when she has a cold, use essential oils for things like headaches, insect bites, or wounds, and drink herbal teas. Whether you are new to the concept, an expert, or somewhere in between, I encourage you to continue learning about these potent gifts from God.

We learn in Scripture that in the beginning of creation itself, God spoke. It was through God's Word that the universe and everything in it came to being. John 1: 1 states, "*In the beginning was the Word, and the Word was with God, and the Word was God.*" Words are powerful. Dr. David Stewart, Ph D. further explains:

AND GOD SAID:

Ezekiel 47: 12

Along the bank of the river, on this side and that, will grow all kinds of trees used for food; their leaves will not wither, and their fruit will not fail. They will bear fruit every month, because their water flows from the sanctuary. Their fruit will be for food, and their leaves for medicine.

AND GOD SAID:

Proverbs 7: 17

I have perfumed my bed with myrrh, aloes, and cinnamon.

"Word is a vibration, a frequency, a consciousness, an expression of energy. When God created the plants by His speaking voice, he imbued them with his Word and his intelligence. This includes the oils of the plants which he intended, from their very creation, to become our medicines when we need healing. This is what is so special about essential oils [and herbs]. They contain power from God's Word. Artificial medicines, made by humans, contain no such power. That is why they cannot heal and never will.... Man-made pharmaceuticals lack the life-force, the intelligence, and the vibrational energy found in healing oils." (*68)

That being said, a common mistake I see, that I encourage you to avoid, is to expect an oil or herb to give you instantaneous results. No one oil or herb will be a "cure all" for what you are dealing with. I see this a lot in the essential oil world especially. "Take X oil for Y ailment." Essential oils and herbs have powerful medicinal benefits, true, but they work best when used in combination with the other concepts discussed in this book. Nothing beats preventative maintenance, good nutrition, quality sleep, physical and spiritual exercise, prayer, and balance for health and vitality. Then, should you have a specific issue that needs extra healing (be it physical, mental, emotional, or spiritual), you can turn to oils and herbs to give yourself a bigger boost in the right direction.

I used to think learning about herbs and essential oils was a bit overwhelming and thought that I would never learn enough about them to really know when and how to best use them. However, a friend once told me that you can't learn about anything overnight. It's consistent learning over time that has a bigger impact. So, since then, I focus on learning at least one herb and/or essential oil each month. After a year, that was 12 herbs and/or essential oils that I was very familiar with and knew well. After 5 years I knew over 60! Granted, there are still hundreds I haven't explored yet, but I now have much more in my arsenal than I did before and these essential oils and herbs have not only benefited me and my family, but my pets and the animals on our homestead as well. Yes, you can use essential oils on kids, pets, and animals; however, I do encourage you to become knowledgeable and well-versed in the essential oil or herb before administering to animals or children.

Essential Oils

Essential oils are mentioned frequently throughout scripture in applications of anointing, medicine, perfume, celebration, and worship. Oils were highly valued, and I'm sure that had something to do with the complexity of the process of extracting them since they didn't have the modern distillation equipment that we do today. Plus, even throughout ancient history, man had a deep understanding of the power of these oils to heal. Biblically, as previously mentioned, there are over 1300 references to essential oils and/or the aromatic plants from which they were extracted. In this chapter, I'll share with you some of the top oils mentioned in the Bible, some history about them, and how they can be used. But what makes them so valuable and so special, what do we need to know about them, and how can we best utilize them for maximum benefit? Well, I'm so glad you asked!

Essential oils are basically the highly concentrated version of the natural oils or resins found in plants. We generally get the oils from the plants through a process called distillation, and the resulting product contains all the characteristic fragrance, the properties of the plant from which it was extracted, and the essence and intelligence of the plant, including its healing properties. Plants possess compounds that contribute to the health of the plant, reproduction, pollination, and protection. These same compounds contain vital living energy ("life energy") that resonates at varying frequencies that interact at varying levels with the cells of our body. Scientists call these compounds "constituents" and have identified over 3000 different constituents of varying amounts and diversity. These constituents, much like the phytonutrients found in fruits, vegetables, and greens that we consume from plants, are still not fully understood. Still, scientists marvel at the complexity and medicinal power of these tiny molecules found in all essential oils.

Scientists further classify the constituents of essential oils into three main categories: Phenols, Monoterpenes, and Sesquiterpenes. Phenols have been proven to be effective at creating conditions in the body where harmful viruses and bacteria cannot live, and more importantly, to clean receptor sites on the cells of the body for improved cellular communication. Essential oils with high levels of phenols include anise, clove, basil, oregano, thyme, and cinnamon. Monoterpenes have been proven to reprogram misinformation in cellular memory (DNA), and they offer a variety of healing properties. Essential oils with high levels of monoterpenes include grapefruit, angelica, frankincense, cypress, galbanum, pine, Rose of Sharon, juniper, spruce, myrtle, hyssop, and peppermint. Sesquiterpenes have been proven to deliver oxygen to the cells, erase miswritten codes in cellular memory, and are powerful at anti-cancer healing. Essential oils high in sesquiterpenes include cedarwood, vetiver, sandalwood, patchouli, ginger, myrrh, spikenard, and black pepper. (*69)

AND GOD SAID:

Song of Solomon 5: 1

I am come into my garden, my sister, my spouse: I have gathered my myrrh with my spice; I have eaten my honeycomb with my honey; I have drunk my wine with my milk. Eat, O friends; drink, yea, drink abundantly, O beloved.

Psalm 45: 8

All thy garments smell of myrrh, and aloes, and cassia, out of the ivory palaces, whereby they have made thee glad.

Due to their small molecular size, and the fact that they are lipid soluble, essential oils quickly and easily penetrate the cell membranes, even if the cell membranes have hardened because of an oxygen deficiency. In fact, studies show that the constituents in essential oils have the ability to affect every cell in the body within twenty minutes of initial contact and then be metabolized like other nutrients. (*63) And the most amazing part is that essential oil constituents only seem to affect the cells that need them!

Many essential oil constituents have properties that are antioxidant, antibacterial, antifungal, anti-infectious, antimicrobial, antitumor, antiparasitic, antiviral, and antiseptic. (*63) Oils can be used for physical concerns, and they are equally powerful in balancing emotional, neurological, and spiritual imbalances. The smells of certain oils like citrus oils, cedar wood, chamomile, or lavender have been proven to uplift the mood, while others like frankincense, peppermint, basil, clary sage, or juniper berry can improve mental clarity.

Essential oil usage can be aromatically (we breathe the aroma, often from diffusing the essential oil), topically (placed directly on the skin...usually with a quality carrier oil or lotion to dilute the potency and avoid sensitivity), or internally (ingested...just be sure to only ingest quality oils that have been certified for internal use. Not all essential oils are created equal and not all essential oils are safe for internal consumption. Only consume essential oils internally under the recommendations and directions of a certified healthcare professional who is well-versed in oils. Essential oils are very potent, and taking them orally can be dangerous).

How you choose to use them depends on the essential oil, the desired results, and the quality of the oil. **Only use high quality oils that are therapeutic grade and certified pure.** In this case, cheaper is definitely not better. There are many reputable brands that carry quality oils. Do your research and choose the best for you and your family. Cheaper oils of inferior quality are often diluted, won't offer the same results, and in some cases can cause more harm than good.

There are hundreds of essential oil varieties and fragrances available on the market, all with qualities to benefit our mind and our body. A few of the essential oils specifically mentioned in scripture include:

Calamus, Cassia, Cedarwood, Cinnamon, Cypress, Fir, Frankincense, Galbanum, Hyssop, Juniper, Myrrh, Myrtle, Pine, and Spikenard.

Probably the best known oils of the Bible are Frankincense and Myrrh, being two of the gifts given to the baby Jesus by the Magi, or Wise Men, from the east. The third gift was gold. Symbolically, these gifts carried great significance.

Gold

Gold was a gift reserved for kings, and a token of their recognition of this child as royalty. Some scholars believe that the gift brought to the baby Jesus was not the *metal* gold, as is often portrayed today, but rather another essential oil or resin, balsam, also sometimes referred to as the Balm of Gilead. This essential oil was so valuable, it was often referred to as "gold", and was used to anoint the kings of Israel. The symbolism of gifting this royal anointing oil, with powerful healing qualities, to the King of Kings is interesting and a powerful message to the people of the time.

Interestingly, Balm of Gilead is found seven times in the Bible and is mentioned in both Genesis and in Revelation. As legend has it, Balm of Gilead, also know by many other names like Balm of Jericho and Balm of Mecca, was a hybrid cultivar of a tree from the same family as Frankincense and Myrrh. However, these trees required the care of a skilled gardener for them to flourish and survive. The extra work was worth it, however, because the resin from the tree was worth more than gold in some areas, particularly for its highly medicinal qualities. Medicinally, the Balm of Gilead was anti-inflammatory, anaesthetic, and had anti-fungal properties. It promoted wound healing and was reported to heal the stomach of a variety of illnesses. Unfortunately, the last tree died around 400 years ago and this healing oil, thought to have been one of the gifts to the baby Jesus, can no longer be found.

Frankincense

Frankincense is one of my personal favorite essential oils, and the perfect gift for the baby Jesus. Frankincense comes from resin from the Boswellia sacra tree, which oozes out and is collected after splitting the trunk. Symbolically, frankincense "is said to have been an acknowledgement of Jesus' priesthood, setting him apart from a typical king. Frankincense was used in the temple routines, burned ceremonially by the priests. It was not native to that region,

AND GOD SAID:

Matthew 2: 11

And when they were come into the house, they saw the young child with Mary his mother, and fell down, and worshipped him: and when they had opened their treasures, they presented unto him gifts; gold, and fankincense, and myrrh.

Leviticus 24: 7

And thou shalt put pure fankincense upon each row, that it may be on the bread for a memorial, even an offering made by fire unto the Lord.

however, so obtaining frankincense from the east was costly. This gift was precious in both meaning and value." (*64) Old Testament accounts also indicate the value of this powerful oil, particularly as an incense, in rituals, and as a medicine.

Health benefits of frankincense are numerous as it is anti-catarrhal, anticancer, antidepressant, anti-infectious, anti-inflammatory, antiseptic, anti-tumor, expectorant, immune stimulant, and sedative. (*65)

I love the smell of frankincense and use it regularly. After my husband's cancer treatment, we have included frankincense in his daily recovery routine (along with diet and lifestyle changes) with amazing results.

Myrrh

Myrrh is referenced more times in Scripture than any other essential oil or aroma, with references in Genesis (37: 25) and in Revelation (18: 13) and multiple mentions throughout the Bible in between with a total of around 156 verses including this powerful essential oil. Myrrh was one of the key ingredients in Moses's holy anointing oil and myrrh was one of the three gifts given to the baby Jesus by the Magi. Some speculate the significance of myrrh as a gift represented Jesus death and resurrection because Myrrh was often used during embalming. However, most likely they offered myrrh for a more practical reason.

Myrrh was highly prized for its medicinal qualities and was often used during pregnancy and postpartum. Myrrh was used after childbirth to prevent or remove stretch marks and reduce anxiety, and it was placed on the baby's umbilical cord to protect the navel from infection. Myrrh could be used to heal cuts, wounds, bruises, coughs, thrush, ringworm, sore throats, chapped skin, and countless other ailments.

Myrrh mixes well with other oils and is considered a synergistic oil because it tends to enhance the qualities of any oil with which it is mixed. On its own, however, myrrh is "antiseptic, supports the immune system, enhances the body's natural defenses, helps sooth the skin, is oxygenating to the body tissues, is mood elevating, creates a sense of well-being, and promotes overall health, vitality, and longevity." (*70) Since Myrrh has one of the highest levels of sesquiterpenes (60%), myrrh is a powerful oil in enhancing oxygen in the cells and repairing damaged cellular memory, making it one of the most effective oils for cancer treatment and supporting emotional balance.

Spikenard

All four Gospels tell the story about a women who anoints Jesus with a very valuable and costly oil from an alabaster jar, found in Matthew 26: 1-13, Mark 14: 1-9, Luke 7: 36-50, and John 12: 1-8. Contained is this jar was a mixture of myrrh and spikenard. Spikenard oil comes from a flowering herb native to the Himalayan Mountains of India and Tibet and had to be imported from there by caravans. To protect this valuable oil, it was often shipped in boxes carved from alabaster or gypsum. It is estimated that the oil poured over Jesus' head and feet would have been valued at that time at around a year's salary.

Why did the woman anoint Jesus with spikenard and myrrh oils? This event is believed to have happened around 2 days before Jesus' arrest. Many scholars believe that the oil was applied as a symbolic preparation for Jesus' coming death. Myrrh, as previously mentioned, was often used during death rituals and embalming. But what about spikenard? Spikenard was often used as a perfume, but the most common use was as a mood enhancer and to reduce anxiety. It is believed that the woman anointed Jesus with Spikenard to help give him strength for the upcoming ordeal of his trial and persecution.

Modern uses for spikenard include supporting healing from allergies, migraines, nausea, emotional calming, and mood elevation. Spikenard is ant-inflammatory, antispasmodic, antibacterial, antifungal, works as an effective sedative, deodorant, and laxative, and as a tonic.

Cassia and Cinnamon

Cassia and Cinnamon are both oils mentioned in Exodus 30: 22-31 as ingredients in God's Holy Anointing Oil. Both cassia and cinnamon come from the bark of the same genus of plants, *cinnamomum.* Both have similar qualities and a similar aroma, with cassia being somewhat stronger and cinnamon being more common and economical. Both are excellent oils for balancing blood sugar, supporting emotional balance, supporting immune system functions, and settling the stomach.

Personally, cassia and cinnamon are some of my favorite scents. I find myself gravitating to them often, however my husband says he doesn't care for their aroma at all. It is interesting how we are all different and respond to oils according to our emotional, spiritual, and physical needs.

AND GOD SAID:

Song of Solomon 4: 13-14

Thy plants are an orchard of pomegranates, with pleasant fruits; camphire with spikenard, spikenard and saffron, calamus and cinnamon, with all trees of frankincense; myrrh and aloes, with all the chief spices.

Revelation 18: 13

Cinnamon, and ointments, and frankincense, and wine, and oil, and fine flour, and wheat, and beasts, and sheep, and horses, and chariots, and slaves, and souls of men.

Other Notable Oils

The Bible mentions many other essential oils and aromas, all with mental, spiritual, and physical healing qualities. Other oils mentioned specifically include:

- **Sandalwood** (also sometimes referred to as Aloes), scientifically found to be antidepressant, antiseptic, anti-tumor, aphrodisiac, astringent, calming, and as a sedative. It was used historically during times of worship to enhance meditation. Medically, sandalwood supports the cardiovascular system, nervous system, and circulatory system. (*71)
- **Cedarwood**, scientifically found to be anti-fungal, astringent, diuretic, sedative, and an excellent insect repellent. This essential oil comes from the wood of the cedar tree, and was cited in 1 Kings 4: 33 as a durable and sustaining wood, used to build Solomon's temple.
- **Cypress**, scientifically found to be beneficial as a lymphatic and prostrate decongestant, supportive to the liver and respiratory system, mucolytic deodorant, and anti-microbial. Medicinally, cypress was also used in cases of excess loss of body fluids. Cypress essential oil comes from branches of the cypress tree, one of the most durable woods found on the earth. Cypress was used to build the doors of St. Peter's Basilica in Rome, and after over 1200 years these doors still show no sign of decay. When my husband and I first got married, we built a log cabin out of cypress. It was amazing wood to work with and I can easily see why scripture mentions it numerous times.

These are just a few of the essential oils mentioned in Scripture. There are hundreds of other essential oils found to be beneficial to our health, not all specifically mentioned, but all equally valuable. A few of my favorite essential oils that bear mentioning due to their diversity of benefits include Lavender, Peppermint, Oregano, and Melaleuca or Tea Tree. I encourage you to talk to a healthcare professional familiar with essential oils, and try incorporating some essential oils into your routine. The oils you start with will depend on your personal needs and preferences. I always find it fascinating how each person can react so differently to the various aromas of essential oils.

Even more fascinating is watching how animals react to essential oils and herbs. Living on a small homestead, we have horses, cows, goats, chickens, ducks, turkeys, dogs, cats, and a bunny. Animals, too, can benefit from the use of essential oils, and unlike their human counterparts, they have a strong natural instinct to what their body needs for healing, both physically and mentally. There is no such thing as a placebo effect when working with animals, and they are very quick to respond and "tell" you which essential oils or herbs they need. It never ceases to amaze me how quickly they respond to the treatment.

I remember one time a couple years ago when we had a very dear horse pass away. He was the solid cornerstone in the herd at 28 years old and had been in the family for almost all of those years. The other horses had a very hard time emotionally adjusting to his passing, showing signs of depression. They went off their feed, started picking fights with each other, and were less likely to romp and play in the pasture. Yes, in case you're not familiar with animals, they all have a deep capacity for emotion. After just one treatment of essential oils, both remaining horses showed almost instantaneous results. For one horse, the preference was lavender essential oil. The other horse gravitated towards peppermint. Overall, it took three days of letting them smell the oils for them to return to normal, but improvement was seen after just the first day. I've seen similar results with all the animals for various issues including wounds, post-partum care, parasite control, and digestive issues.

We also regularly use essential oils in our home as a chemical-free and non-toxic cleaning option, and we use essential oils in our garden, orchard, and vineyard for natural and organic pest control.

One final quick thought on essential oils. Earlier I mentioned how essential oils resonate at a certain frequency of vibrational energy, which contributes to the power of the essential oil on the body. Interestingly, in a study done by Dr. Bruce Tainio, of Tainio Technology in Cheny, Washington, the frequency of several essential oils was measured and monitored under various conditions. In his study, Dr. Tainio found that negative thoughts actually lowered the frequency of the oils by 12 MHz while positive thoughts raised the frequency of the oils by 10 MHz. This in and of itself is quite interesting and shows how powerful our thoughts can be! Yet, Dr. Tainio took his study one step further. Adding prayer with positive thoughts raised the frequency of the oils by 15 MHz. We all know how powerful prayer is! Combine prayer with essential oils and the combination is incredibly powerful. Biblically, oils were often applied as anointing, during deep prayer. Moses says in Deuteronomy 7:13 that God will bless the oil of the righteous person. We can now see through scientific measurements, how this is literally the case. (* 72)

AND GOD SAID:

Isaiah 44: 14

He heweth him down cedars, and taketh the cypress and the oak, which he strengtheneth for himself among the trees of the forest.

Luke 11: 42

Woe to you Pharisees, because you give God a tenth of your mint, dill, cumin, rue and all other kinds of garden herbs, but you neglect justice and the love of God.

Herbs (and Spices)

The term "herbs" is generally used to reference parts of plants, including leaves, grasses, seeds, stems, stalks, roots, flowers, berries, and nuts, which are used for their culinary or therapeutic and health-promoting properties. The more I learn about herbs and experiment with them in my cooking, my gardening, and my healthy lifestyle, the more I love them. Herbs and spices offer flavor to our dishes, with underlying benefits of phytonutrients and "living energy" to support our health. Whether it's through an herbal tea, tincture, infusion, poultice, or simply adding them to a dish, herbs and spices bring color to an otherwise blank white page in our diets.

It seems like there is an herb for just about any taste, issue, complaint, or problem. Herbs can be sweet, sour, salty, bitter, or savory. They can cool the body or warm it up. Some herbs help the body with detoxification. Others help balance minerals and keep you regular. There are herbs to support every major organ and body function, and even herbs to help reverse gray hair! Just as with essential oils, I recommend seeking the guidance of a professional who is familiar with herbs to help guide you on getting started with which herbs might work best for you and your specific concerns. The purpose here is to point out the power of herbs and encourage you to start incorporating more herbs and spices into your lifestyle. Entire books and educational courses are available for those interested in diving deeper into the world of herbs, how to prepare them, and how to use them.

Some of my favorite culinary herbs include:

Allspice, Basil, Bay Leaf, Caraway Seed, Cardamom, Chia Seed, Chili Powder, Chives, Cilantro, Cinnamon, Clove, Coriander Seed, Cumin, Curry, Dill, Fennel, Fenugreek, Garlic, Ginger, Lavender, Marjoram, Mint, Mustard Seed, Nutmeg, Nutritional Yeast, Oregano, Paprika, Parsley, Pepper, Rosemary, Sage, Thyme, Turmeric, Vanilla

Medicinal herbs that I always have on hand include:

Aloe Vera, American Ginseng, Ashwagandha, Bee Pollen, Calendula, Cayenne Pepper, Chamomile, Comfrey, Dandelion (leaves and roots), Echinacea, Fo-Ti (He Shou Wu), Holy Basil, Lemongrass, Maca Root, Red Raspberry Leaf, and Stinging Nettle

There are many herbs listed throughout Scripture, and the people of Biblical times used herbs on a daily basis. Herbs were common place in medicine, cosmetic ointments, aromatics, fumigation, religious rituals, embalming, and cooking. (*73) Although we don't necessarily need to use herbs today for embalming, you too can use herbs in all the other ways listed. And, the best part about herbs is that they are easy to grow, economical to purchase, and fun to use.

Many herbs come from beautiful plants that brighten up your landscape, like calendula, chamomile, and lavender. Others, like dandelion and stinging nettle, are considered weeds. But both dandelion and stinging nettle are a couple of my favorite herbs that I consume almost daily. Dandelion supports the digestive system, acts as a liver tonic, and helps the body detoxify. Stinging nettle is high in iron, a mineral that I find myself often deficient. I used to suffer from extreme fatigue caused by low iron levels (anemia) and commercial supplements would cause me to become constipated. Since adding stinging nettle to my morning tea, I haven't had any symptoms of anemia or chronic fatigue!

Another favorite is comfrey. Comfrey is a beautiful, broad, fuzzy-leafed plant with tiny purple flowers. A seemingly otherwise boring plant, comfrey has powerful healing capabilities for cuts and wounds. In fact, my herb mentor once told me to be sure the wound is good and clean before you put any comfrey on the wound, because it will close up so fast it might just seal any dirt or debris in the wound! On the homestead, we have comfrey planted throughout the pastures for the animals. Most of the time, they leave them alone, but every so often you'll see an animal go to town chowing down on those plants. Interestingly, they especially love to eat the comfrey right after giving birth. I guess the animals know that this amazing herb has the ability to help their bodies heal and recover.

Medicinal herbs are so interesting, and God gave us these plants to help our bodies heal. Some medicinal herbs can cause reactions, especially if taken together with pharmaceutical drugs. Be sure to use caution and seek professional advice when trying new herbs, especially if you are taking medication, pregnant, nursing, or offering them to children. That being said, approximately 100,000 people each year die from the adverse reactions or side-effects of pharmaceutical drugs. Deaths, or even hospitalizations, due to herbal (or essential oil) reactions or side-effects are so rare that no specific statistic could even be found. (*74) I did find a few statistics on hospitalizations from commercial dietary supplements, but that's not what we are talking about here.

AND GOD SAID:

Luke 13: 9

It is like a grain of mustard seed, which a man took and cast into his garden; and it grew, and waxed a great tree; and the birds of the air lodged in the branches of it.

Exodus 12: 8

And they shall eat meat, roasted with fire, and unleavened bread; and with bitter herbs they shall eat it.

Herbs are a natural gift from God to help us heal in ways our bodies are more readily able to identify, assimilate, and process, often with no side-effects or reactions.

Speak with an herbal specialist in your area for additional assistance in determining the best herbs for your situation and the recommended application and dosage, if needed. Enjoy the amazing and powerful "life energy" found in the leaves, stems, flowers, and roots of these wonderful herbal gifts from God.

Spiritual Significance of Essential Oils and Herbs

Spiritually, essential oils and herbs played a major role throughout Biblical history. The most common spiritual reference to essential oils is in reference to anointing. For most of my life, I never really understood what it meant to be anointed with oils, and the significance behind this act. This confusion may in part be contributed to the multiple customs associated with anointing as referenced in scripture. "Anointing" had personal, medicinal, and religious traditions, all of which consisted of a mixture of essential oils with a carrier oil. In some cases, the anointing oil was over 80% essential oils, and the one being anointed had large quantities of oil poured over his or her head or feet (much different than the dab of anointing oil used in many churches today).

Personal anointing was a custom during biblical times to pour olive oil and essential oils over one's head, face, and body as a form of cleansing and deodorizing. The oils help soothe the skin from the sun, dust, and dry heat.

Medicinal anointing is mentioned throughout scripture in both the Old and New Testament. Anointing with oils was used as a form of healing. In fact, one account of the origin of the practice of anointing points to ancient shepherds. Lice and other parasitic insects would often burrow into the wool of the sheep, where they would sometimes transmit diseases and kill the sheep, particularly if they got into the ears. So, the resourceful shepherds figured out that pouring certain essential oils and a carrier oil like olive oil would make the wool slippery and would protect the animal from the pests. From this, anointing became symbolic of blessing, protection, and empowerment. (*75)

Religious anointing signified God's blessing or call on that person's life. In many cases, it represented God's blessing on the calling for kings, but could also

171

represent God's blessing on a calling to be a prophet, a teacher, or other "divinely chosen" profession.

In Exodus 30: 23-24, God gave Moses the specific formula and instructions for the "holy anointing oil" which included Myrrh, Cassia, Cinnamon, Calamus, and Olive Oil. This holy anointed oil was to be used to anoint not just the priests but the tabernacle and all that was inside. This included the Ark of the Covenant, the alter, the pillars, the floor, the tools and utensils. Interestingly, the compounds found in the formula would have made this oil very effective at disinfecting, with anti-bacterial, anti-viral, and anti-fungal properties.

Today, the spiritual significance of anointing with oil can represent God's blessing for a spiritual calling we may be facing, prayers for the blessing of healing, as a symbol of worship and obedience, and celebration for answered prayers. Anointing oil can also be used on homes or articles that may possess demonic presence, to cast them away.

Some may balk at the last, feeling that we don't have demonic spirits anymore. Personally, however, I have faced them many times throughout my life. On one instance, my husband and I had just moved into our first home together. I was home by myself one night when I was faced with the clear presence of a demon. Only through prayer, and the help of my pastor coming out to anoint the house with oils, and proclaiming his leaving by the power of Jesus name, did the demon leave and not return.

Anointing oils, when prepared according to God's direction, carry powerful cleansing and healing properties. Use them prayerfully and if needed for your life.

AND GOD SAID:

Exodus 29: 7

Thou shalt take the anointing oil and pour it upon his head and anoint him.

Theologenic Diet
List of Essential Oils and Herbs

The following is a summary of some of the primary essential oils and herbs found in Scripture or recommended for their healthy qualities. This list is by no means complete, as there are thousands of varieties of plants, herbs, and oils that can be beneficial to your health. This list is designed as a starting point to help you in making healthier choices. I encourage you to continue to learn about Essential Oils and herbs, and to experiment to find the ones that work best for you.

Essential Oils (be sure to select only pure, therapeutic grade essential oils from a reputable source and dilute with a carrier oil for best results. Only ingest under the supervision of a professional.)

Basil, Bergamot, Black Pepper, Calamus, Cassia, Cedarwood, Cinnamon, Clary Sage, Clove, Copiaba, Cypress, Eucalyptus, Fennel, Fir, Frankincense, Galbanum, Grapefruit, Hyssop, Juniper, Lavender, Lemon, Lime, Melaleuca (Tea Tree), Myrrh, Myrtle, Oregano, Peppermint, Pine, Rose, Rosemary, Sandalwood (Aloes), Spikenard, Thyme

Culinary Herbs (fresh or dried)

Allspice, Basil, Bay Leaf, Caraway Seed, Cardamom, Chia Seed, Chili Powder, Chives, Cilantro, Cinnamon, Clove, Coriander Seed, Cumin, Curry, Dill, Fennel, Fenugreek, Garlic, Ginger, Lavender, Marjoram, Mint, Mustard Seed, Nutmeg, Nutritional Yeast, Oregano, Paprika, Parsley, Pepper, Rosemary, Sage, Thyme, Turmeric, Vanilla

Medicinal Herbs (used fresh, dried, as an infusion, as a tincture, in a tonic, in teas, in poultices, mixed with lotions, soaps, or salves, or in an herbal steam)

Aloe Vera, American Ginseng, Ashwagandha, Bee Pollen, Calendula, Cayenne Pepper, Chamomile, Comfrey, Dandelion (leaves and roots), Echinacea, Fo-Ti (He Shou Wu), Holy Basil, Lemongrass, Maca Root, Red Raspberry Leaf, and Stinging Nettle

Chapter Summary:

God has given us a wide array of plant compounds that offer powerful medicinal and nutritional value when included in a healthy lifestyle, particularly in the form of essential oils and herbs. Essential oils and herbs contain high concentrations of "life energy" to support our bodies physically, emotionally, and spiritually. Essential oils and herbs, when used correctly, are safe and effective without the common side-effects of pharmaceuticals. Consult a professional aromatherapist or herbalist in your area for specific varieties that might be best for you.

Action Steps:

1. Start using culinary herbs in your everyday dishes. Experiment to find the flavors you like best and the preparations you prefer. Become familiar with which culinary herbs add heat (like cayenne, cinnamon, and black pepper) and which herbs are cooling (like mint, dill, and cilantro).
2. Try adding herbal teas to your routine, whether it's a invigorating tea blend in the morning like yerba mate, spiced chai, or peppermint, or a relaxing tea blend in the evening to help you wind down, like lavender, chamomile, lemon balm, and passion flower.
3. Become familiar with essential oils, particularly the top oils of the Bible like Frankincense and Myrrh, and popular essential oils like lavender and peppermint. Consult a professional if needed, and consider adding essential oils when needed to your routine.

Notes:

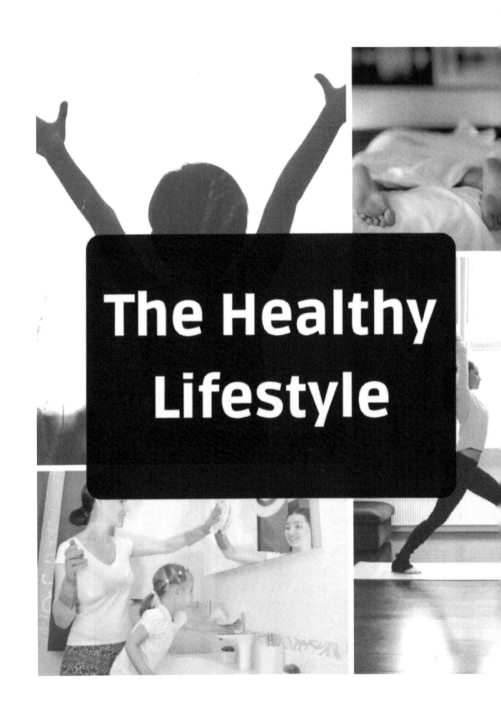

The Healthy Lifestyle

Chapter 13: Fasting, Cleansing, & Detoxing

The first step to "change" and improving your life, your energy, and your health is knowledge. In the previous chapters, I went into great detail about the core components of what a healthy diet according to God's plan would consist of. We went into what to eat, and what not to eat, so that you can shift your thinking about food and make better choices. Now that you have the knowledge about food and "life energy", and hopefully started putting that knowledge into action, we can start looking at the other key aspects of life that God defines for us in order to have optimum health. What we put into our bodies and our minds as fuel is the foundation to health. Once your foundation is established and you have put your new knowledge into action, it's time to start building the walls and the roof of your temple body. The walls are your *lifestyle* and the roof is your *mind, thoughts, and attitude.*

The next several chapters will shift from food guidelines to lifestyle, and how you may be impacting your health by other choices in your life besides the food you eat. In this chapter, we will start by looking at fasting, cleansing, and detoxification.

Most likely, if you've been eating according to common cultural practices, your body is loaded with toxins. When your body gets exposed to too many toxins, chemicals, and foreign substances, the body naturally will do what it needs to protect the vital organs like the heart and the brain. Those toxins then get shoved into fat cells to be dealt with at a later time, theoretically when your body can catch up on the toxic overload. Unfortunately, if we continue to live in toxic environments and throw more toxins at our bodies, the clean up crew can never quite catch up. At some point, the toxins build up so much that you start to experience symptoms like constipation, weight gain, excessive body odor, blood pressure issues, and headaches. If left unchecked, the immune system becomes compromised, leaving the body exposed for diseases and illnesses to set in.

Think about it this way. If every day you came home from work, or school, or whatever you usually do in a day, with a large bag (or two) of trash, and left it in your house. Pretty quickly the house would change, right? Even with a cleaning crew coming in once in awhile to clean for you, it wouldn't take long for the trash to over-run the place. At first, you might try sticking bags into closets or in your

AND GOD SAID:

1 Peter 2: 5

You also, as living stones, are being built up as a spiritual house for a holy priesthood, to offer up spiritual sacrifices acceptable to God through Jesus Christ.

1 Corinthians 6: 19-20

Do you not know that your bodies are temples of the Holy Spirit, who is in you, whom you have received from God? You are not your own; you were bought at a price. Therefore honor God with your bodies.

basement to get that clutter and stinkiness out of the way, but eventually you would run out of room and those bags would be overflowing every closet, cabinet, and shelf. Eventually they would fill the rooms, making comfortable living impossible. You may try using scented sprays to mask the stench of the trash, but that never really fixes the problem, only temporarily covers the smell. Your comfortable sanctuary quickly becomes a place of stress and aggravation. Your sleep becomes affected, due to the constant smell and the annoyance of bags everywhere. At some point, rodents, insects, and other pests start moving in, drawn to what they perceive as prime real estate.

Not a pretty picture, right? You wouldn't do that to your house, your home, your sanctuary; so why are you doing it to your body? Every day that you bring "home" trash and toxins, your body has to deal with it, and it doesn't take long for the trash to start getting backed up, causing all kinds of issues. Has your trash built up enough that you can't sleep, don't feel well, and the pests (diseases) have moved in? Just like your home, sometimes you need to do a deep clean. Even when you are not bringing trash home everyday, the dirt and grime will naturally build up in your home, requiring some cleaning attention. Your body is the same way. Depending on how toxic your body is right now, how many years of toxic build up you may be dealing with, and the ability of your body to clean, will determine how you go about proceeding.

Note: If you're currently dealing with a major health issue, be sure to work closely with your professional healthcare provider. Depending on your level of toxicity, your liver, adrenals, thyroid, kidneys, and digestive system may be over worked and not functioning at the optimum level. Mass media and marketing has created a hype about detoxing, particularly to get you to buy their products. I will discuss detoxing shortly, and I am a big supporter of detoxing your body, however detoxing should never be done until your cleaning crew is up to the task. Consider our house example. If your house is so full of trash bags that you can barely walk anymore, and your cleaning crew is so tired and overworked from hours and hours of constant attempts to bring order back into the chaos, if you were to walk in one day and say, "I've had enough, I want this house cleaned from top to bottom, starting right now, and we're not going to rest until every trash bag is gone," what do you think your cleaning crew would do? Most likely they would quit and walk out on you.

That's why we started first with gradually introducing your body to healthier food choices and adjusting your diet, chapter by chapter. If you've been following

178

along with the action items offered after each chapter, then your cleaning crew has been given a bit of a vacation from dealing with so much new toxins coming in every day. Little by little, your body has been slowly regaining some balance. But before we start looking at detoxing, we need to give your poor clean up crew a bonus. Why not give them a raise, along with the rest, so that they will more enthusiastically and energetically go back to work on the deep, spring cleaning we are about to ask them to do? I am referring to Fasting.

Fasting

Fasting was a common practice throughout biblical traditions, and Jesus often fasted. Fasting, is simply removing food or a type of food for a period of time, for the sake of some spiritual purpose. There are many types of fasting including Absolute Fasting (removing all food and drinks for a period of time), Liquid Fasting (removing all foods for a period of time, consuming only water, vegetable juices, and green juices), and Partial Fasting (removing certain foods for a period of time).

In the Bible, we see many examples of fasting, often during times of challenges and need for deep spiritual enlightenment or intervention. During fasting there are often two benefits:

1. The first, is that by eliminating foods or types of foods from our diets, we are basically rebooting our digestive system, much like rebooting our computers or phones (someday this statement will date the writing of this book). During a fast, our digestive system gets a much needed break, hormones can reset, enzymes can get produced, and toxins can get flushed out.
2. The second benefit, is that when entered into prayerfully and by replacing food with communion with God, fasting deepens our connection to the Holy Father. I have heard countless testimonials of miraculous healing, breakthroughs, answered prayers, and divine intervention during times of fasting.

The tradition of fasting has become a rare thing in today's culture. Many Christians are aware of fasting, but few practice fasting on a regular basis, other than the short-term "mini" fast done each night while they sleep...only alleviated the next morning when they break the fast (Breakfast). But, in Matthew 6: 16, Jesus doesn't say to his disciples "if," but "when you fast."

AND GOD SAID:

Psalm 35: 13

I humbled my soul with fasting; and my prayer returned into mine own bosom.

AND GOD SAID:

Daniel 1: 12-13

Please test your servants for ten days: Give us nothing but vegetables to eat and water to drink. Then compare our appearance with that of the young men who eat your royal food, and treat your servants in accordance with what you see. (NIV)

Fasting from food or a type of food for a period of time shifts your focus from the worldly self to the spiritual self and allows a deeper connection with God. This shift from physical food to spiritual food can often ease that spiritual hunger you may be experiencing and not even know it on a conscious level.

Although it may sound simple enough, the reality of the world, our flesh, and the devil will often conspire against us by introducing all sorts of complications that make abstaining from food and focusing on God instead, difficult. The first time I fasted, I had to overcome the temptations of a catered business meeting, family get-together, kid's birthday party, and church bake sale! Should you prayerfully decide to fast, here are a few tips and guidelines to get you on your path:

Set Your Objective

The important first step in fasting is knowing why you are fasting and what you hope the fasting will accomplish. Is it healing, spiritual renewal, divine guidance, or God's grace to handle a difficult situation? Ask the Holy Spirit to offer clarity for your objectives, that they follow God's plan for you.

Start Simple

Pray about which type of fast you should undertake. As stated earlier, there are many different types of fasting. The direction you choose will depend on personal preference and what God puts on your heart. Before you fast, decide how long you will fast and what type of fast. Be sure to take into consideration how those around you, like family members, may be affected by your fast. Communicate with them and get their support.

A great starting point is a one or two day liquid fast. This is a short-term fast in which you only consume water, fresh vegetable juices, and green juices. The benefit of this fast is that the liquids help with feelings of hunger, and will help keep your blood sugar balanced for energy.

Another great option for fasting is a Daniel Fast. The Daniel Fast consists of consuming only those foods outlined in the book of Daniel as outlined in verses 12-13: "Please test your servants for ten days. Give us nothing but vegetables to eat and water to drink. Then compare our appearance with that of the young men who eat the royal food, and treat your servants in accordance with what you

180

see." Most contemporary versions of the Daniel Fast include vegetables, fruits, nuts, seeds, grains, beans, and legumes, healthy oils, and herbs. Cut from the diet are all processed foods, sugar, and animal products like eggs, meat, and dairy. If you've been following the principles outlined in this book, you're pretty much already following the Daniel Fast food guidelines anyway. You'll just be eliminating any animal products you currently may be consuming and adding the spiritual element. You can do a Daniel Fast for ten days or 21 days.

Plan Before Starting

Once you have prayerfully decided to fast and chosen the type of fast you will perform, you'll want to plan how you will fill the time in spiritual feasting when you would otherwise be physically feasting. Plan to takes some time in prayer and meditation, serving others, or communing with God. I heard a pastor say one time that "Fasting without a purpose and a plan is not Christian Fasting; it's just going hungry." Have a clear picture going into the fast what you are looking for from the fast, how you plan to go about it, and what prior preparations need to be done. Part of your preparations include preparing yourself spiritually. The foundation of fasting is repentance, so spending some time reflecting on, confessing, and asking for forgiveness for your sins is a crucial part of preparing for your fast.

Prepare Yourself Physically

Depending on the type of fast you choose, you may want to consult your healthcare provider first, especially if you are taking any prescription medication or a chronic illness. There are some cases where a person should only fast under the supervision of a healthcare professional.

Start your Fast

Enjoy the process. While you are fasting, turn your focus to God and enjoy the deep communion time with your Heavenly Father. Enter into the fast with an expectant heart (Hebrews 11: 6). Meditate on the attributes of God, His love, compassion, grace, faithfulness, power, and wisdom. Ask God to fill you with His Holy Spirit and follow where He leads you. And most importantly, do not underestimate the power of spiritual opposition. Satan will often pull out all the stops during a fast. Keep your eyes on the Lord and remember that Satan doesn't bother with people he already has control over. He only attacks those he fears the most. You got this! Because our God is sovereign and bigger than anything Satan can throw at us.

AND GOD SAID:

Hebrews 11: 6

And without faith it is impossible to prease God, because anyone who comes to him must believe that he exists and that he rewards those who earnestly seek him. (NIV)

Isaiah 1: 16

Wash! Cleanse yourselves. Remove your sinful deeds from my sight! (NIV)

Once you have completed your fast, ease back into foods slowly and avoid heavy or fatty foods for the first couple days to give your digestive system a chance to readjust. Enjoy the feelings that come with completing a fast. Some experience deep peace, joy, lightness, fulfillment, or a sense of completeness. Regardless of your outcome, give thanks and praise for the experience. Try to make it a regular part of your life to include some type of fast during times when you need deeper spiritual connection or intervention. Sometimes that intervention may be for loved ones who need healing or God's help. Other times it may be for a community or church. Keep an open heart and listen to the Holy Spirit which will guide you through your fast and put it on your heart when you need to fast again.

Cleansing

Another way to support your body is by cleansing. "Cleansing" is defined as making something clean, ridding something or someone of unpleasant, unwanted, or defiling substances, or freeing someone from sin or guilt. The Bible often references cleansing and it is important to cleanse regularly. Cleansing can refer to personal hygiene, internal cleansing, and how we clean our personal environment.

Personal Hygiene

Keeping ourselves clean is an important part of health. This includes regular bathing, with attention to body, hair, and teeth. My parents did a really good job of raising me and I thought I was doing a really good job on my personal hygiene. It wasn't until recently, however, that I came to learn and realize how product choices I had been making over the years was harming my body. As I mentioned in the chapter about essential oils, the skin is the largest organ of the body and absorbs whatever is put on it surprisingly fast, which goes right into the bloodstream. This little known fact is one of the great powers of using essential oils topically, yet at the same time can be extremely detrimental when we use commercial soaps, lotions, perfumes, shampoos, hair dyes, and other products that are loaded with harmful chemicals. The cosmetic and body care industries date back thousands of years, to even before biblical times, yet the ingredients have drastically changed over the years. How can we actually be cleaning our bodies when we are using products that contain harmful toxins that are absorbed through the skin into the body, only to have to be dealt with by the liver and kidneys?

Luckily there are some companies out there who do pay attention to their ingredients and offer healthier choices that aren't made from things like parabens, aluminum, isopropyl alcohol, quats, SLS, and petroleum-based oils. Check out the Resources section for some examples of companies who don't use harmful chemicals in their products.

Deodorant is one example. Many products on the market are both deodorant and antiperspirant. However, antiperspirants restrict the body's production of sweat. Sweat is a natural cooling mechanism and also one of the ways your body eliminates toxins. By restricting this ability, your body is not able to function the way God designed it. Additionally, we apply deodorant directly under our armpits, right where one of the body's lymph nodes are located. The lymph nodes act as filtration systems and are crucial to the cleansing of the body internally. When lymph nodes get clogged or backed up, illness and even cancers can occur. Switching to a product that is a deodorant only, made from more natural ingredients, is recommended.

Another big switch I made was hair care. Little did I know or understand in my youth how damaging all those shampoos, conditioners, gels, sprays, and dyes were to my hair. Much like pharmaceuticals that have side effects that create the need for more pharmaceuticals, hair products often have side effects that cause the need for other products. Even after countless studies have shown the lathering agents, quats, and other synthetic ingredients to be carcinogenic and potentially cancer causing, companies continue to use them. And consumers continue to buy them.

I was guilty of this for years. I would buy a bottle of shampoo by the smell, or the price, or the convenience, or what my stylist recommended. And after my hair started falling out, I was told that it is normal to loose hair every day; not to worry. When my hair became thin, frizzy, and listless, I just added more products. And worst of all, I just suffered through the burning and discomfort to my scalp every time I had my hair colored, thinking there were no other options. I was totally amazed when I finally saw the light and switched to a natural hair-care product line that worked for me. My hair quickly became soft and vibrant again and my scalp felt so much better. I didn't have to suffer through the pain that always came with coloring.

AND GOD SAID:

Leviticus 15: 13

And when he that hath an issue is cleansed of his issue; then he shall number to himself seven days for cleansing, and wash his clothes, and bathe his flesh in running water, and shall be clean. (NIV)

Psalm 51: 2

Wash me thoroughly from mine iniquity, and cleanse me from my sin.

I saw amazing results when I switched to a natural skin-care line and mineral cosmetics, too. The skin is a reflection of what we feed our bodies, our hydration, our stress levels, how much sun exposure, and what products we use. For healthy glowing skin, be sure to follow the food guidelines outlined in this book, drink enough water, protect your skin from the sun, and use products that include God-made ingredients instead of man-made ingredients.

And that goes for your oral hygiene too! Did you know that the majority of commercial toothpastes on the market actually contain sugar? And the other ingredients are often toxic when ingested, so why are we putting this in our mouths...and in our children's mouths? Baking soda based toothpastes without those harmful chemicals are more effective, particularly those with added essential oils like myrrh, clove, and peppermint. Don't forget to floss, too!

Environmental Cleansing

Part of supporting a healthy lifestyle is reducing the toxic and chemical exposure in your environment. Granted, we live in a toxic world, and we will never completely eliminate all the toxins around us, but there ARE things we can do to improve our environment. First, our home should be our sanctuary; the place we go to relax, unwind, enjoy family, and live a fulfilled life. How safe is your home and does it support a healthy lifestyle? Did you know that at the time of writing this book, there are approximately 85,000 chemicals regulated under the United States Toxic Substances Control Act (TSCA) but the Environmental Protection Agency has only tested a fraction of these for human toxicity! In one study, the Environmental Working Group tested the toxicity of newborns. In this study they analyzed the cord blood of newborn babies for toxins. The results were astounding. They found an average of 287 chemicals in the newborn cord blood, of which 180 were cancer causing, 217 were toxic to the brain and nervous system, and 208 cause birth defects or abnormal development in animal tests! (*77) Here are a few things to look at in your home environment to see if you can make it less toxic:

- *How clean is the air in your home?* Whether you live in a house, an apartment, or a tent, you need clean air to breathe, as discussed in chapter 2. Modern construction attempts to create tight homes with less air flow while under the impression that it makes the home more energy efficient. Where this might be the case, if the home is too air tight, the air inside can become stagnant. A recent study published in the journal "Science of the Total Environment" found that the air indoors is often more polluted than the air outside. (*76) Older homes, or newer homes with moisture issues, have increased risk of mold and bacteria in the air, too. Some things you can do is open your windows on nice days to encourage fresh air circulation, change out the air filters regularly in your air conditioner, and run air purifiers, particularly in the bedrooms. Avoid the use of scented candles, as many brands actually add toxins to the air. Opt to diffuse essential oils instead if you want some scent in the air.

- *How toxic is your laundry?* I was reading a recent report that claimed fabric softeners as one of the highest sources of harmful toxins in the home. I'm not sure how true that is, but it makes sense, especially when you consider that those little fibers on the dryer sheets are made of toxic chemicals, which end up in the fibers of the clothes. Those clothes sit against your skin all day, and as we've discussed, the skin absorbs those toxins into the bloodstream. Instead of fabric softener, consider switching to dryer balls. Dryer balls are balls of natural wool yarn that you can easily make yourself, and are effective at fluffing and softening the clothes while they dry. If you miss the scent from the commercial softeners, add your favorite essential oils instead. Laundry soap is another source of toxic fragrances and synthetic cleaners. Check out the Recipe section for our favorite homemade laundry detergent or switch to a non-toxic brand. Not only will it be better for the health of your family, but will reduce the toxins added to the environment! A definite win-win!

- *How toxic are your cleaning products?* A couple years ago, an F5 tornado touched down in a town about 50 miles from my home. Hundreds of homes and businesses were destroyed. The clean-up from that disaster took months before any rebuilding could take place. But, after the electrical wires were removed and the debris was cleared away, the biggest challenge came from an unexpected source. All those homes contained thousands of bottles of chemicals in the form of household cleaners, pesticides, chemical fertilizers, and other toxic household items, many of which ended up breaking open and seeping into the ground and into the water supply. It was at that time that I took a hard look at how many toxic substances I had in my home and used on a regular basis, often unnecessarily. Since then, I have eliminated 99% of the chemicals I was using in my home. Instead of harmful chemicals in my cleaning supplies, I use micro-fiber cloths and natural products. Instead of pesticides, I use essential oils. Instead of chemical fertilizers, I use compost. My home is still clean, and in many cases the natural products

AND GOD SAID:

James 4: 8

Draw nigh to God, and h will draw nigh to you. Cleanse your hands, ye sinners; and purify your hearts.

185

AND GOD SAID:

Matthew 6: 16

Whenever you fast, don't be sad-faced like the hypocrites. For they make their faces unaddractive so their fasting is obvious to people. I assure you, they've got their reward.

work even better than the chemical counterparts. Plus, I have peace of mind knowing that I am not exposing my family, my friends, or my pets to toxins or chemicals that could harm them.

- *How toxic are the people with which you surround yourself?* Toxicity can be physical but it can also be mental. Negative energy affects our thoughts and our thoughts affect our moods and our actions. Be aware of the people in your life and whether they are neutral, building you up, or tearing you down. Those who are consistently adding negative energy are not contributing to your health. Negative energy can also come from the music you listen to, the social media you engage in, and the "entertainment" you choose to watch. Be mindful, pray for guidance, and avoid negative energy whenever possible.

Note: These same principles also apply to your work environment, although you may not have as much control over the air or the chemicals used. When possible, be the spark that ignites positive change in your workplace, and do what you can. If change where you work is not an option, creating a safe haven in your home becomes all the more crucial for your health.

Detoxing

Detoxing and cleansing are terms often used interchangeably, so to avoid any confusion, let me explain the difference. "Cleansing" is where you remove something or several things that may be contributing to your issues. "Detoxing" is where you go even deeper to allow your body to remove toxins that may have been stored for some time. There are several types of detoxes you can do, including a full deep detox where you detox the body, and isolated detoxes such as a skin detox, organ detox, foot detox, etc.

I am a big believer in detoxing and find it especially beneficial. However, since detoxing is more of a deeper "spring cleaning" of the body, I don't advise doing a full deep detox until your body can handle it. Toxins that have been stored need to be reprocessed through the liver and kidneys to be eliminated so be sure these systems are up for the task. Isolated detoxes are fantastic, however, and can be done pretty much anytime. If you are at all concerned, always consult with your healthcare professional prior to starting any detox.

Skin Detox

Because the skin is the largest organ of the body and one of the ways the body eliminates toxins (through sweat), an occasional skin detox is wonderful. Natural elements like activated charcoal, Bentonite clay, and oatmeal have amazing qualities to draw out impurities and toxins from the skin. I love regularly doing a detox mask on my face, my underarms, and under my breasts. When I am feeling especially decadent, I'll soak in a bath with dead sea salts, or Himalayan salts with Bentonite clay and essential oils to detox the skin on my whole body. I then follow up with a good natural lotion to moisturize. You can adjust the essential oils added based on what may be specific health concerns. For example, adding lavender will help you sleep, eucalyptus is great for respiratory issues, or frankincense and myrrh for just about anything inflammatory.

Organ Detox

There may be times when you have a certain organ or area of the body you want to pinpoint for a deeper detox, such as the liver, kidneys, gall bladder, or adrenals. In cases such as this, it is recommended you work with a professional healthcare provider who can guide you in the specific herbs and foods that will be best for your situation. In most cases, an organ detox consists of eliminating certain foods for a period of time and adding certain botanicals that are known to help with the organ in question. Don't attempt an organ detox without the guidance of a professional, especially if you have chronic issues.

Foot Detox

Feet are a fascinating part of the body. They take such a beating in the day, and serve us well. The bottoms of the feet contain what are called "reflexology points," which are points that correspond with various organs and other parts of the body. These points are generated because the foot is what is considered the end of the body's meridians, or energy flows. Detoxing the feet can not only benefit the foot, but the whole body as well. A few benefits of a foot detox include removing of toxins, reduction of swelling, calming to the body, boosting the immune system, possible balancing of blood sugar, and boosting cardiovascular health. You can detox the feet with a charcoal and/or Bentonite clay mask, ionizing foot bath, foot scrubs, soak in Epsom, Dead Sea, or Himalayan salts, or through detox foot pads.

AND GOD SAID:

Mark 9: 29

And he said unto them, this kind can come forth by nothing, but by prayer and fasting.

1 Corinthians 7: 5

Do not deprive each other except perhaps by mutual consent and for a time, so that you may devote yourselves to prayer and fasting.

Probiotic Detox

One of my favorite isolated detoxes is a probiotic detox. This consists of consuming probiotic-rich, living foods like kombucha, kefir, cultured vegetables, kvass, and yogurt to infuse the gut micro-biodome with as much beneficial bacteria as possible. The gut is the center for the digestion, the immune system, hormones, emotions, and brain function. The more we can support the gut, the better we will feel and the more efficiently our body will perform. Of these, kombucha in particular, is the star when it comes to supporting the body at detoxing. In fact, kombucha has been found to be effective at aiding the body with eliminating heavy metals from the system! Kombucha has also been a powerful tool for cancer patients who have undergone radiation and chemo-therapy, to detox the body from the residual effects of the therapy. Kombucha is delicious, easy to make, and one of my personal favorite "super foods."

Other Great Methods of Detoxing Safely

Other than food elimination, adding herbs, consuming more probiotic-rich foods, and applying masks or salt soaks, there are some wonderful ways to support your body in eliminating toxins for a health and healing. Here are some of my favorites:

- *Infrared Sauna:* Any time your give your body the chance to sweat, you accelerate its ability to remove toxins. Infrared saunas use dry heat that relax the muscles and trigger the body to detox. Drink lots of water after time spent in a sauna.
- *Massage Therapy:* Who doesn't love a good massage? Massage therapy is not only relaxing, but when done properly, encourages the body to release toxins stored in the muscles and fat. Massage therapy can be combined with essential oils and relaxing music for the combined effect of stress reduction, relaxation, and detoxification. Also be sure to drink lots of water after a massage session to help your body hydrate and flush the toxins.
- *Colon Hydrotherapy and Enemas:* Remember that your body is only capable of removing toxins a couple of ways, namely sweating, through the breath, through urination, and through defecation. It is very important to have regular bowel movements. Newborn babies, who generally have pure digestion that hasn't been corrupted by toxic foods, fill their diapers many times a day. Ideally, we should be having a bowel

movement after every meal; at a minimum, at least once every day! It has been estimated that the average overweight American is carrying around an extra 20 pounds just in fecal matter. I know we're getting a little graphic here, but it's important to understand that God designed our bodies to efficiently use the maximum energy from the food we eat and then eliminate the waste. If you find yourself constipated or otherwise not having regular bowel movements, you might consider consulting with a professional colon hydrotherapist. He/she will assist you in balancing your colon flora, and gently cleansing any compacted fecal matter that may be stuck in your colon. Another option is to perform an enema to gently flush the colon. Consult your healthcare provider for recommendations.

Fasting, Cleansing, and Detoxing are ways you can support your body to optimize your health. I often hear comments after a fast, cleanse, or detox with testimonials of more energy, better skin, better sleep, more mental clarity, fewer headaches, fewer seasonal allergies, better love life, and an overall increased feeling of happiness and peace. Although there is no way of knowing your results until you try it for yourself, these healthy habits are worth incorporating into your routine.

Note: Depending on your level of toxicity, you may feel a little worse before you feel better. Know that this is normal. Just like when you clean your house and sometimes it looks worse before it looks better, once you start attacking those toxins, it may feel worse before it feels better. Take heart and don't give up. The temporary discomfort will be worth it in the long run! And God will help you through it all!

189

Chapter Summary:

Even when you eat completely healthy, our bodies are bombarded every day with toxins that need to be identified, processed, and then either stored or eliminated from the body. Over time, if the exposure to these harmful toxins becomes more than our body can easily handle, health issues will start to develop. To avoid toxic overload, support the body the way God taught us through regular fasting, cleansing, and detoxing.

Action Steps:

1. Prayerfully consider partaking in a fast, either a liquid fast, a Daniel Fast, or other fast that works for you. Draw near to God through deep meditation and prayer during your fast and listen to the words God puts on your heart during your fast.
2. Look at the toxins in your immediate environment. How are you affecting your body and the health of yourself and your family through the chemicals found in your home? Consider replacing toxic products for natural, non-toxic products for laundry, cleaning supplies, cosmetics, hair care, body care, sprays and scents, pesticides, and fertilizers. Check out our Resource section for products we have researched and found worth recommending.
3. Consume more probiotic-rich, living foods like kombucha, kefir, cultured vegetables, kvass, and yogurt to support your gut.
4. Get a massage, sit in a sauna, or consider a colon cleanse to further support the body in eliminating stored toxins.

Notes:

Chapter 14: Sleep & Rest

And on the seventh day, God rested. Yes, even God rests, as indicated in Genesis. Rest is a crucial part of physical, mental, and emotional health, because it is when we are resting that our bodies are able to shift gears from conscious activities, and instead focus on healing, cell regeneration, and growth. Rest to restore and repair!

But unfortunately, all too often, we find that much-needed sleep and rest alluding us. Our modern lifestyles have created the perfect storm of cramming too much into our days, with the emphasis on what we can accomplish and how much we can get done rather than priorities of God, family, and taking time for yourself. For years I was guilty of this and as a result, I was stressed and not sleeping. A couple years ago, it was not uncommon for me to wake up in the middle of the night for some reason...and then my thoughts would take over, swirling like a whirlwind through my mind. I would lie there, staring at the ceiling, trying to fall back to sleep but lists of what needed to be done, conversation replays, emotional concerns, and overwhelm would keep me from my much-needed slumber,
at least until about 30 minutes before I was supposed to wake up, at which point I would finally fall into that desired deep sleep. Only to be suddenly awakened all too quickly by that blaring alarm!

Have you ever had nights like that? Either you have trouble falling asleep, or at some point in the night you wake up and the brain kicks into overdrive, thoughts take over, and there's no getting back to sleep, seemingly no matter how hard you try! It's a frustrating feeling, and unfortunately one that if not addressed, can have serious impacts on your health.

I found myself facing nights like this way too often, and it was starting to become a problem. I couldn't seem to get a good night's sleep, and as a result I was tired during the day, dealing with brain fog, irritability, and reduced productivity. I knew this wasn't good for me, but what could I do?

We all know how important sleep is for us. Doctors will tell you to get at least 8 hours of sleep every night, but do you know why they say to get a minimum of eight hours? Getting enough sleep is crucial because it is during sleep that our body shifts its focus from working, thinking, digesting, and other activities, to growing (children), healing, cleansing, and rejuvenating. Sleep is the only time

AND GOD SAID:

Genesis 2: 2

By the seventh day God had finished the work he had been doing; so on the seventh day he rested from all his work.

Psalm 55: 6

Oh that I had the wings of a dove! I would fly away and be at rest.

your brain has to detox, because the brain doesn't have lymph nodes or sweat glands.

But, for those of us balancing work, family, and activities, eight hours of sleep (and even more than that for children) seems like a hilarious number! How are we supposed to get 8 hours of sleep when not only do we have too much on our plate for the hours in the day, but we find ourselves waking up in the wee hours of the morning, staring at the ceiling, our brains rapidly firing away, while we listen to the annoyingly peaceful breathing of our spouse slumbering deeply next to us?

When I was a kid, it seemed like I could sleep just about anywhere. My parents were amazed at how quickly I would fall asleep and how deeply I would sleep anytime I was in a vehicle for any length of time. Once asleep, I was out like a light and we used to joke that a tornado could go by and I wouldn't hear it. Sleep, when I was young, was easy. As I got older, sleep became more difficult. By the time I was 35, I found I was rarely getting a full night's sleep. I had a terrible time getting myself to fall asleep, and when I did I often would toss and turn, then wake up several times throughout the night. Most nights, if I woke up in the middle of the night, I would immediately start thinking of all the things on my "to do" list and find myself several hours later still trying to fall back to sleep, much like the scenario previously described. As a result, I was tired all the time. I found myself turning to caffeine at times for a quick boost and craved sugar in the afternoons. My health suffered and it created a vicious cycle. I desperately needed a good night's sleep and the temptation was to turn to medical intervention. I needed to make some changes so I could be human again. I was losing hope.

But, believe it or not, it *is* possible to sleep again like when we were children, and by following a few simple tips, you can kiss your insomnia good-bye for good! Here are a few changes I made, after research, prayer, and God's guidance that worked for me... (and backed by science), so you too can enjoy a deep, relaxing, and much-needed rest:

Nutrition

Believe it or not, nutrition plays a significant role in how well we sleep. If you have been following the principles outlined in this book, you most likely are already seeing improvements to your sleep quality. Our body needs optimum nutrition to function properly and that includes rest. The most important considerations when filling your plate to help you rest are:

- Cut the processed. Processed foods contain little to no nutritional value and also contain lots of sugar and/or salt. This adds stress on the body including stress on the adrenals, liver, and kidneys.
- Cut the sugar. Sweets treats are great on the palate but they are generally digested quickly, causing a short-term boost of energy followed by a crash. Our bodies are thrown into that horrible cycle of highs and lows that will affect our natural ability to relax.
- Avoid caffeine after 3 p.m. Caffeine is a natural substance found in some foods in small doses like tea and chocolate, but in larger amounts in foods like coffee and soft drinks. Caffeine stimulates the central nervous system, and is a popular remedy to increase alertness. Too much caffeine, however, has deep affects on the body including increased risk of headaches, rapid heartbeat, muscle aches, heartburn, irritability, and confusion. Chronic overuse of caffeine has also been linked to fertility issues, high blood pressure, increased risk of osteoporosis (caffeine prevents calcium absorption), anxiety disorders, and even certain cancers. Caffeine is considered a drug, and has addictive qualities, and withdrawal symptoms. And because it is a stimulant, caffeine disrupts the body's natural ability to relax and fall into that deep sleep needed for healing. Be aware of how much caffeine you consume and avoid caffeine too close to bedtime so your body has time to recover for the stimulating effects before it is time to sleep.
- Add magnesium. An estimated 75% of Americans are magnesium deficient. Magnesium aids in stress reduction and rest. Taking a magnesium supplement, or using a magnesium lotion on your feet right before bed can work wonders not only on sleep but help with other issues like constipation, hypertension, and boosting the immune system.
- Don't eat before bed. During sleep, our bodies are working hard at cleansing, healing, and balancing. We were not designed to efficiently perform both digestion and cleansing at the same time. If you tend to get those late night food cravings, go for herbal teas, a green juice, or a small amount of a healthy fat like avocado. Some experts recommend not eating anything at least two hours before settling in for the night. I had a holistic doctor tell me one time that the body was designed by God to function most efficiently around the sun and the seasons. She said to follow nature in our daily habits, including waking early with the sun and never consuming foods in the dark (when the sun is down).

AND GOD SAID:

Hebrews 4: 9-11

There remains, then, a Sabbath-rest for the people of God; for anyone who enters God's rest also rests from their works, just as God did from his. Let us, therefore, make every effort to enter that rest, so that no one will perish by following their example of disobedience.

Exodus 33: 14

The Lord replied, "My Presence will go with you, and I will give you rest."

Herbs and Essential Oils

Herbs and essential oils, as previously discussed, have incredible nutritional and medicinal values and our bodies can easily assimilate them. Certain herbs and essential oils are particularly beneficial for rest, stress reduction, and sleep. My favorite "Sleep Time Herbal Tea" can be found in the Recipes section of this book. It includes herbs like lavender, chamomile, and valerian root. Essential oils like lavender, frankincense, ylang ylang, vetiver, spikenard, and chamomile have sedative properties that can help with sleep. Inhalation through aromatherapy or topical applications give the essential oils direct access to the brain through smell, relaxes tense muscles, and calms the mind.

Turn Off the Technology

Technology is wonderful. I love how much these various gadgets make life seem easier (or do they?...but that's a topic for a different day...). But despite all their wonderful uses, like entertaining us, staying connected with friends, organizing our days, and informing us of world events, the blue light radiating from our phones, computer screens, tablets, and televisions is interfering with natural triggers in our brain that it is time to sleep. Turn off the technology at least one hour before bed. Instead of that technology, take some much needed down time before turning out the lights by soaking in a relaxing bath, reading, or other relaxing activity you enjoy that doesn't involve a screen.

Grounding

Speaking of technology, we live in such a technological world that we are constantly surrounded by energy from cell phones, computers, tablets, televisions, microwaves, and all the other electrical appliances needed for our "comforts". These are great, and I wouldn't want to go without them, but they do add stress to our bodies through the invisible 'radiation' and positive ions emitted.

A few years ago, a group of Swedish 9th grade students performed an interesting experiment that got worldwide attention from their results. They observed that if they slept with their mobile phones next to their beds near their heads at night, they often had difficulty concentrating at school the next day. To determine the effects of technology on health, they devised an experiment using seeds. In their study, they placed six trays of garden cress seeds into a room without radiation, and six trays of garden cress seeds into another room next to the WiFi routers. In their experiment, and subsequent similar experiments, the seeds placed near the devices all either were completely dead or hadn't grown. The seeds planted in the other room, away from the routers, all thrived. (*78)

To avoid these harmful effects on your body, especially when sleeping, keep all technology out of the bedroom and don't keep your phone on the nightstand next to your bed. Some studies show that during sleep, you want to have at least eight feet or more between technology and your body. Ideally, they should be in a different room. Other studies show that walking outside barefoot for about 10-15 minutes, or using grounding devices such as an Earthing Mat, will also help balance the body, counteract the effects of technology, and improve sleep. I saw a big difference in my sleep when I started using an Earthing Mat under my feet while sitting at my computer. Himalayan Salt Lamps added to your environment also can help diffuse the effects of the harmful ions emitted.

Routine

Try setting up a normal bedtime routine and especially endeavor to go to bed and wake up around the same time each night/morning. I know for many of us that can be a challenge, especially when we have kids...but supporting your natural biorhythms is a must. Even if it's just for a short time while resetting your body clock, try to develop a regular schedule. Included in that schedule might be a nice warm bath or shower, read a book for a few minutes, go through your hygiene routine, and prayer.

Darkness

Although you wouldn't think that darkness would make a significant difference in your sleep, studies show that total darkness stimulates the body to produce melatonin, a natural hormone that makes you sleepy. When your body senses light it will produce less melatonin and when it's dark you will produce more. Light can throw off your body, even if it's a soft glow from a nightlight, the glowing numbers on your digital clock, or the light coming from the hallway or bathroom. If you live in the city where there are streetlights, consider getting black-out curtains or wear an eye pillow. Avoid taking commercial supplements that contain melatonin. Some studies show that taking melatonin inhibits your body's natural ability to produce it, creating a possible dependency issue.

AND GOD SAID:

Psalm 4: 8

In peace I will lie down and sleep, for you alone, Lord, make me dwell in safety.

AND GOD SAID:

Matthew 11: 28-30

Come to me, all you who are weary and burdened, and I will give you rest. Take my yoke upon you and learn from me, for I am gentle and humble in heart, and you will find rest for your soulds. For my yoke is easy and my burden is light.

Get Comfortable

Ok, I know that may seem obvious...but...if you're not sleeping well, consider your sleeping environment and adjust if needed. Check the room temperature and adjust if possible. For most, a cooler bedroom temperature is more conducive to better sleep. Is your mattress and/or pillow in need of some updating? What noise levels are you dealing with and do you need a fan or some other "white noise" to cover up background distractions? Take inventory on anything you may need to change in your sleeping environment to help with your comfort and consequently your sleep quality.

Prayer

Stress is a main deterrent to a good night's rest, and the best remedy for stress is to turn to God in prayer. Cast your troubles on Him, trust and have faith that He will guide you through, and focus on your blessings. Spending time with God at the end of the day, before you retire, with a sense of gratitude will greatly impact your sleep and the nature of your dreams.

Take Time for Yourself

Part of resting is taking time to recharge. Even our technology needs rebooted once in awhile, and we are no exceptions. Most of this chapter I am focusing on tips for better sleep, yet it is also important to consider the value of rest and taking time for yourself. Take your day of rest, as God did after creation. Take breaks, take vacations, take time to dream, take a moment to redefine your purpose. Rest is cornerstone to health and will support your whole being including physically, mentally, emotionally, and spiritually. Don't underestimate the power of a good recharge and reset that comes with taking some time for yourself.

Final Thoughts on Sleep and Rest

In recent years, medical professionals and organizations like the National Sleep Foundation have defined sleep, along with nutrition and exercise, as one of the three pillars to health. Although it may take some conscious determination to change old habits, both routine habits and mental habits, making it a priority to get sufficient deep sleep can benefit you through better health, better mental clarity, better balance, and a more positive outlook. Full disclosure, getting enough sleep is still my biggest personal challenge, but by making it a priority, setting myself up for success through better habits and routines, and turning the rest over to God, I do much better than I used to, only rarely staring at the ceiling in the middle of the night. When I do, it's usually because I slipped back into old habits that day. And, it continually gets easier to keep the good habits going! So take heart and give these tips a try. What do you have to loose, other than your insomnia?

AND GOD SAID:

Psalm 23

The Lord is my shepherd, I shall not want. He makes me lie down in green pastures, he leads me beside still waters, he refreshes my soul. He huides me along the right paths for his name's sake. Even though I walk through the darkest valley, I will fear no evil, for you are with me; your rod and your staff, they comfort me.

Chapter Summary:

Getting enough rest is one of the most important things you can do for your health next to nutrition and exercise. When you sleep, your body is finally able to focus on restoring and repairing. If you are not getting enough sleep, look at your habits, your environment, and your stress levels to see what changes can be made to support sleep.

Action Steps:

1. Make it a priority to get at least 8 hours of good sleep each night.
2. Remove technology from the bedroom, particularly any WiFi devices next to the bed.
3. Don't eat and avoid caffeine at least two hours before bedtime.
4. Take time for yourself to relax. Spend time with God in prayer and turn everything over to Him.
5. If you are still having trouble sleeping, try an herbal tea and/or essential oils to support a good night's sleep.

Notes:

Chapter 15: Movement & Exercise

God designed our bodies to move, and staying active is one of the key pillars to health. When my husband was recovering from major surgery a couple years ago, the physical therapist told us about a study done on the importance of movement for better recovery. He told us that in clinical studies they have found that patients who stay in bed following surgery have higher risks of muscle loss, heart and lung capacity reduction, increased risk of complications, and longer recovery times. He stressed the importance of pushing through the pain and moving, because without it, permanent damage could occur. So even after a fourteen hour surgery, they had him up and walking the very next day!

Even when we are not recovering from surgery, movement is important. Exercise is key to a strong heart, good circulation, muscle tone, weight control, hormone balancing, metabolism, energy levels, deep sleep, skin health, mental clarity, and an overall sense of well being and happiness.

When we exercise, core areas of the body experience physiological and biological changes. A few examples include:

Muscles: Our muscles use glucose and ATP for contraction and movement. To create more ATP, your body need extra oxygen. During exercise, breathing increases and your heart starts pumping more blood to your muscles. The more you use your muscles, including the heart muscle, the greater the stamina, endurance, and strength.

Heart: Your heart is included in the muscle group, but is a unique muscle in that its primary job is circulating blood throughout the body. During exercise, the heart rate increases to supply more oxygenated blood to the muscles. The more you exercise, the more efficiently your heart becomes, allowing you to work out longer or harder. New blood vessels form, which helps balance blood pressure.

Lungs: During exercise, your body requires much more oxygen; as much as 15 times more oxygen than when you are at rest). As a result, your breathing rate increases to accommodate for this increased need for oxygen. The more you exercise, the greater the lung capacity. As mentioned in chapter two of this book, every cell in our body needs oxygen to thrive. Through movement, we encourage that needed cellular oxygenation.

AND GOD SAID:

Philippians 4: 13

I can do all things through Christ who strengthens me.

1 Timothy 4: 8

For while bodily training is of value, godliness is of value in every way.

Joints and Bones: At some point in our adult lives, we achieve peak bone mass, after which begins a slow decline. Exercise, however, can help the body maintain healthy bone mass as we age. The more inactive we are, the more brittle our bones become due to their porous nature. Movement and exercise, along with a healthy diet (particularly foods like bone broth that contain collagen, gelatin, glucosamine, and condroiten), are the best preventative measures for joint or bone problems.

Brain: Exercise increases blood flow throughout the whole body, including the brain. This increased blood flow and oxygenation helps the brain function better. Have you ever noticed after a workout that you feel more mentally focused, more creative, or more engaged? Interestingly, some studies show that exercise promotes the growth of brain cells, particularly in the hippocampus, the part of the brain that boosts memory and learning. Essentially, exercise encourages your brain to work at its optimum capacity by causing the nerve cells to multiply, strengthens their interconnections, and protects them from damage.

Also, during exercise, a number of neurotransmitters like endorphins, serotonin, dopamine, and glutamate are triggered. These neurotransmitters are well-known for their role in emotions and mood control. As a result, exercise is one of the best natural remedies for depression, insomnia, and stress.

"According to a 2012 study published in the journal *Neuroscience,* the "secret" to increased productivity and happiness on any given day is a long-term investment in regular exercise. And a little each day appears to go further than a lot once or twice a week." (*79) The most important word here is "regular". Without making it a conscious habit every day to get your body moving enough to increase your heart rate and maybe work up a bit of a sweat, your health may be suffering.

Now, if you are reading this and you have a consistent routine established, pat yourself on the back and give yourself some kuddos. Congratulations and way to go! If you're not, don't beat yourself up about it. Too often, we know what is best for ourselves and then succumb to feelings of guilt or self-deprecation when we fall short of our own expectations. For years I struggled with this, knowing how important it was for me to exercise, yet so often, time got away from me and I didn't get a workout fit into the busy schedule of work, kids, events, and responsibilities. Then I would feel guilty and bad about myself for not getting it done. But those whispered negative thoughts in my head were definitely not rom God. If you find it hard, like I did at first, to make it a regular habit to exercise, here are a few tips that might help you get started.

Start Small

Movement and exercise don't have to be marathons to be beneficial. When my husband was recovering from surgery, it was one slow and difficult walking lap around the nurse's station. Today, he could do that in about 10 seconds, but at the time it was a very challenging feat. Start small and within the limitations of your current abilities. Then, slowly continue to build on what you have done to push yourself just a little bit longer and/or a little bit harder.

My daughter was wanting to get ready for the "Track and Field Fun Day" at school. This is a play-day event every year at the school where the kids compete in friendly track events. She was a bit frustrated, because she said she couldn't run very far or very fast. So, her dad and I encouraged her to run on our driveway (we live in the country, with a long private drive) to practice. Her dad coached her to run as far as she could before she had to stop and walk. Then do the same the next day and see if she could run a little bit farther. After just a couple weeks of this, she was running up and down the driveway several times before she needed to stop. Over time she was able to build her stamina, strength, endurance, and speed.

So often, we fall into the trap of wanting things quickly and without effort. But health, strength, and endurance, are things that come over time and with perseverance. No matter where you are now, just start at the level that is comfortable for you, and then build from there.

Make it Fun

Exercise shouldn't be work. Part of the problem I had with fitting exercise into my routine was that I was going about it all wrong and looking at it like another task", or "duty" I had to do. When I shifted my thinking to defining exercise as the time in my day that I get to unwind and have fun, everything changed. I found I looked forward to my workouts and it became easier to fit it into my day. Exercise doesn't have to be jumping up and down in front of your TV watching skinny models cheer you on... unless, of course, you find that fun and enjoyable! For me, I found it more beneficial to go for power walks, ride my horses, swim, or take my bike down the trail. During colder months, I like to get on the treadmill while I listen to inspirational videos. Find what works for you, that you

AND GOD SAID:

Proverbs 24: 5

A wise man is full of strength, and a man of knowledge enhances his might.

2 Timothy 2: 5

An athlete who runs in a race cannot win the prize unless he obeys the rules.

look forward to doing, and stick with it until it becomes a habit and a regular part of your routine.

Find a Buddy

For some people, they are fine with scheduling a workout and sticking with that schedule, but for others, especially at first, it may be beneficial to find a workout buddy. Invite a friend or loved one to join you. Not only will you have fun sharing the experience, but you now have an accountability partner to help keep you on track. And you can be a blessing to them as well, by offering encouragement along the way. If you have young kids, encourage them to join you in some of your workouts. You set the example for their future habits, and it can be a fun adventure to do together.

The key to having a workout buddy is to make the promise to yourself up front that should your workout buddy ever bail on you, that you won't give up. Find a new buddy or keep on going. You never want to let anyone else dictate your success or stand in the way of your goals.

Set a Routine

During biblical times, the people didn't need to worry about finding time to exercise because they walked everywhere they went, labored hard to grow and cook their food, and spent most of their days moving. Today, things have changed a little bit. I heard Tony Robbins once describe our modern world very well by saying we live in a world of boxes. We wake up on a box, drive to work in a box, to sit in a box, talk on a box, and type on a box. Then we come home to a box, eat out of a box, while we stare at a box to unwind. I wonder if that's where the concept of "thinking outside the box" comes from? During all this "box" time, we get complacent in sedentary lives, eating unhealthy foods, and then wonder why we are tired, sick, can't sleep, and have no energy!

Instead, shake things up a bit and get out of the box world. Stop eating out of a box, start taking time to move. At first you may have to set a routine until exercise becomes a habit that you look forward to, and stick to your plan. Over time, you will find your body adjusting and then craving that time you spend moving. As a result, it gets easier and easier, and your body will feel better and better.

Take Breaks

If you are already blessed with a lifestyle where you are constantly moving, then you understand the importance of taking breaks so your body can rest occasionally. Conversely, the same holds true for those of us with more sedentary lifestyles and jobs that don't involve as much movement. If you are in a lifestyle where you sit at a desk, or don't move much, it is just as important that you take regular breaks to MOVE as it is for the physical job to take breaks to REST! Stand up, go for a short walk, stretch, breathe deep, climb some stairs, do some jumping jacks, dance, or anything else that engages your heart, lungs, and muscles. Experts say that you should stretch or walk at least three to five minutes for every 90 minutes of sedentary time. If you do, not only will you feel better and support your health, but you will be more productive as well!

So don't let those excuses or that guilt hold you back any longer. Just start somewhere and go from there. You'll find it gets easier as you go, especially as you start to feel the benefits regular exercise has to offer. Listen to your body, listen to the Holy Spirit within you, and enjoy the process. If I can do it, I know you can too! You got this!

AND GOD SAID:

Isaiah 40: 31

...but those who hope in the Lord will renew their strength. They will soar on wings like eagles; they will run and not grow weary, they will walk and not be faint.

Chapter Summary:

Our bodies were designed by God to move to be most effective and maximize health, and this applies to all ages. Movement encourages better circulation and oxygenation, and supports the body physically, emotionally, mentally, and spiritually. Exercise doesn't have to be a strenuous or long workout. Any movement that raises the heart rate for at least 15-20 minutes has been proven to be beneficial to health.

Action Steps:

1. Make it a priority to get some exercise in every day, where you are able to stretch your muscles, increase your heart rate, and breathe deeply. Consult your healthcare provider if needed to recommend a program that is best for you.
2. Make exercise fun and set up your routine! Gradually increase intensity and/or length to continue to improve your strength, stamina, and endurance.
3. Be sure to stretch before and after your workouts, and drink lots of water to stay hydrated, particularly during and after the workout.

Notes:

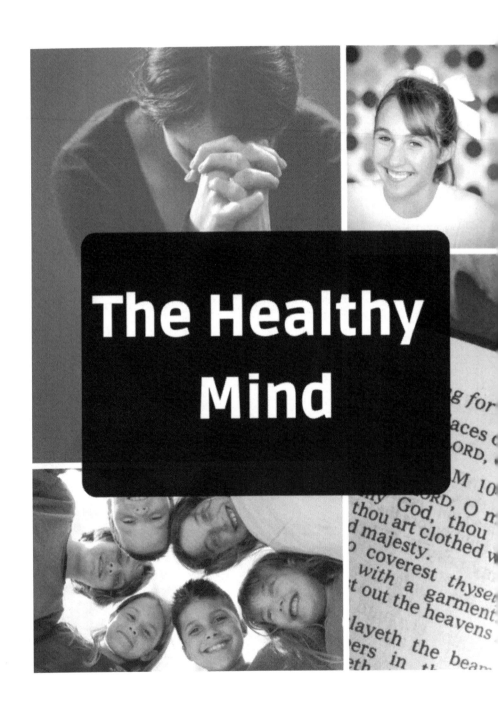

The Healthy Mind

Chapter 16: Healing, Prayer, & the Power of Your Mind

Everything you have read so far in this book was to educate you on the specifics of what God says about diet, health, and nutrition in such a way that you can more fully grasp and logically reason how these concepts will fit into your life. Nothing I said so far, however, will be of any use to you unless you combine putting the concepts into action, along with conscious thought, prayer, and faith. I believe that this is a main reason why so many diets fail. Not only do they not follow God's principles, but they don't teach you how to combine your physical actions, your physical choices, and your left-brain conscious logical thought with your right-brain sub-consciousness, emotional self, and core beliefs.

Now that you have read through the facts presented so far, your logical brain may have accepted or rejected the ideas, concepts, and studies discussed. You may be analytically and consciously ready to make some changes to develop new habits. Without addressing the subconscious, however, old habits will too quickly take back over and once again you will find yourself in that vicious cycle of trying a new diet, falling off the wagon, feeling guilty, then convincing yourself it doesn't work and moving on to the next big idea that comes along.

The truth is that the patterns we have established are deeply ingrained and are connected to our emotional selves. And, it is our emotions that more strongly dictate our actions, try to take over our thoughts, and influence our outcomes. This concept applies to all areas of our life, not just food and health. It is only through recognizing that you are ultimately the master of your thoughts, the creator of your emotions, and a child of God with the Holy Spirit residing within you, that you will break through those old habits and start to find the strength and perseverance, through faith, to make positive changes for the better in your life.

How many times have you heard stories of people who beat the odds, surprised the doctors, or pulled themselves out of seemingly impossible situations? These stories are inspirational and encouraging, and your story could be one of them. Science, through recent technology that allows the measuring of energies, has found that during prayer, a higher level of vibrational frequency is reached. Science has also proven that higher levels of vibrational energy influence healing,

AND GOD SAID:

Isaiah 55: 8-9

God decides who will be healed, while still living in our earth, and who will be healed by passing through to eternal life. For my thoughts are not your thoughts, neither are your ways my ways. As the heavens are higher than the earth, so my ways are higher than your ways and my thoughts higher than your thoughts.

both physically and emotionally. Throughout the Bible, God gives us guidelines to follow, such as love, forgiveness, gratitude, empathy, serving others, and righteousness; all of which resonate a higher energy level when we experience them. But, because we are not perfect, and because we all sin, we tend to continually find ourselves falling into old habits that are of this world. That's why we need God's love and His forgiveness. That's why we need ways to continue to grow and learn, either through a church family or other support groups. Changing your lifestyle to follow God's guidelines on health is no different than following God's guidelines on all the other aspects of the Bible.

Old habits, as they say, die hard. Why? Because they have become intertwined with how you perceive yourself, your emotional response, and your sub-conscious. When we try to form a new habit, the logical left-brain goes to war, essentially, with the sub-conscious right-brain. In order to break through, you need to form a new sub-conscious reality. The great thing about our sub-conscious, though, is that the sub-conscious has a hard time differentiating between real thought and imaginary thought. This is why visualization and prayer are so important. Follow these steps to changing your inner sub-conscious, so you can win the battle against those underlying core habits and create new healthier habits defined by God.

1. Seek out the Holy Spirit within and ask for intervention on your behalf. Pray for strength, wisdom, perseverance, and fortitude. Cravings and addictions are powerful forces, and anyone who says you just need more will-power is misleading you. Will-power is a finite resource. It will only take you so far. When you stumble, do your best to avoid succumbing to guilt and self-blame. Turn to God with a grateful heart and push forward with determination to continue to do better. I believe in you and God's got your back.

2. Start each day with words of affirmation and recite verses outlined in this book. Words are powerful and by saying them out loud, you tap into both your conscious and sub-conscious mind. Be careful to avoid negative self-talk. Instead, focus on an affirmation statement like, "I am a blessed child of God, and I am Healthy, Strong, Energetic, and Worthy of God's Abundant Blessings." Always make affirmation statements in the present tense, not future tense, as if it has already happened and embodies your current state.

3. Think about what it is you want to achieve. Is it healing? Deeper relationships? Better sleep? Energy? Peace? Visualize yourself as if you have already achieved what it is you want and think about the person you need to be, the actions you need to take, and the mindset you need to create, as if it has already happened. In every miracle Jesus performed, the people had to DO something (with faith), to achieve their miracle. Never did Jesus ever walk up to someone and simply heal them. They had to ask for it in faith, and then perform some act such as getting up, touching his garment, washing, etc. Ask, Do, and Visualize as if it is done...all in faith.

4. Recognize that you are the master of your thoughts and emotions. They do not control you, you control them. Be the Master. When you notice thoughts and emotions trying to take over your actions in a way that is not helpful or positive, recognize that you are in control and shift your perspective. Have you ever seen a couple arguing about something, their emotions heated...when suddenly the phone rings or someone knocks on the door? What happens? The emotions are quickly and suddenly switched to address the new situation or person. You can do this in every situation, but it does take some practice. Build the skill of taking control of your thoughts and emotions, turning to God for guidance.

5. Develop a deeper relationship with God through prayer. Take time to listen for His voice, not just ask for things. Come to Him in praise, worship, and thanksgiving. I grew up going to a conservative protestant church and most of my life I didn't really know HOW to pray. I remember asking my mom one time what it truly means to pray. She patiently explained that prayer is our way of talking to God on a deep level.

The Bible says to pray unceasingly, meaning we praise God through prayer throughout the day, not just before meals or before bedtime. We don't need to ask God to be with us, as He is always there. Rather we take time to acknowledge His presence, His generosity, and His abundance in our lives. Prayer is our time to go to God on behalf of others, and to seek wisdom, patience, and strength. Prayer, like any other form of communication, develops and deepens as we mature in Christ. As small children, we recite simple memorized prayers. But as we

AND GOD SAID:

James 3: 13-15

Is any one of you in trouble? He should pray. Is anyone happy? Let him sing songs of praise. Is anyone of you sick? He should call the elders of the church to pray over him and anoint him with oil in the name of the Lord. And the prayer offered in faith will make the sick person will; the Lord will raise him up.

Psalm 34: 19

A righteous man will have many troubles, but the Lord delivers him from them all.

mature, we can eventually deepen into rewarding two-way communications where we hear His voice and feel His presence.

I once heard it explained this way in a sermon at my church. Prayer is a word or series of words spoken to God through the Holy Spirit. In this sermon, the pastor said that he believes that prayer is a way for us to learn to speak like God speaks. For example, in Genesis, God's first prayer was in the form of three simple words, "Let there be..." Those three basic words can then be shortened into one word: Amen. When we say "amen," it is our way of saying "let it be so." To pray like God prays, we must speak like God speaks, and begin and end with "Let there be..." Then, we need to turn our prayers and petitions over to God in faith, knowing that he has heard our prayers.

6. Be patient. Have patience with yourself and with God. Know that God is always in control and He will never forsake you. Even when you don't always feel His presence, He is there. If we pray for something and don't immediately get what we want, know that God hears all our prayers and answers them in His own way, in His own time, and in a way that will most benefit us.

7. Have grace with those around you. Not everyone in your inner circle will agree with what you are doing in changing your lifestyle. Granted, I would love to see a mass movement of people who will see how our culture and our modern lifestyles have changed drastically, and not in ways that support a healthy Christian life. But until that day happens, recognize that you may not get support from some of those people closest to you. Just as with any of God's lessons, the best thing we can do is to pray for them, focus on God, and set an example for them. Over time, through God's grace, when they see the changes in you, they too may come around, God willing.

When my mom found out she had cancer, she went to her pastor to seek out comfort, support, and prayers for healing. When she wasn't cured, her pastor told her she didn't have enough faith. It was a devastating blow for her to hear that, when she knew deep in her heart that wasn't true. Even though that pastor had good intentions, the lesson in recounting this experience is that even those who love us deeply can't possibly know everything about us that God knows. If we allow others to

212

influence our thoughts and actions more than God, then we are allowing the world to control us. So, have grace for those around you. Love them, forgive them, and pray for them. In so doing, you will draw nearer to God and find greater comfort, which ultimately leads to a deep peace and joy that can only come from God.

8. That being said, find a like-minded support group if possible. Start a Theologenic study group in your church (see www.TheologenicLife.com for details about our study group resources), join our online community (www.TheologenicDiet.com), or share this book with friends or family who are interested. We are social people by nature, and having the support of others, to bounce ideas off of, to share recipes, and to ask questions is invaluable, especially when we are just getting started.

We live in an information age, where we can pull out our phones and get answers to just about any question, but how do we know which answers are accurate? How do we know what to listen to when multiple answers conflict in their advice? With prayer and communion with the Holy Spirit, God will guide you to the best answers that work for you and your situation.

n Romans 8: 31, we read, "If God is for us, who can be against us?" I find great peace in this verse and have a framed version of it on my desk so I can see it every day. The truth is, God is always for us, but too often it is I, myself, who is my biggest enemy standing against myself. How many times have I let fear, self-doubt, feelings of unworthiness, or negative self-talk get in the way of my relationship with God, my relationship with others, and my success or achieving my goals? If this sounds like you, make it a point to get out of your own way.

Fear is an important emotion designed to keep us safe; yet at the same time, too much fear can keep us stagnant, restricting our growth. Self-doubt, unworthiness, or negativity are tools of the devil, designed to hold us back from achieving our divine purposes. It took me two months to get started writing this book, because I let those inner thoughts hold me back. But, had I not moved forward in faith, only God knows how many people I would not have had the opportunity to help with this message. But even if it is just one person; even if that one person is you, who I was able to touch in a positive way, through the words of this book, then all the tears, effort, and time would be worth it. It is my hope and prayer that you embrace the fear and discomfort, see yourself as the beautiful and amazing child of God that you are, and experience the joy, peace, and abundant health God wants you to have.

AND GOD SAID:

Romans 8: 31

If God is for us, who can be against us?

Notes:

Chapter 17: Putting it All Together

Throughout the pages of this book, I have introduced quite a few concepts about diet, nutrition, health, and lifestyle choices that may be completely new to you. The transition for me and my family was not an overnight occurrence and in full disclosure, we still struggle daily with the temptations of the world. We are not perfect in our food choices, just as we are not perfect in how will live our daily lives. I am a sinner, but I do my best, repent, seek God's counsel, guidance, and forgiveness, and move on. I do my best to arm myself daily with the armor of God and the sword of the Spirit, continually seeking greater wisdom and understanding. At least now, I have more knowledge when it comes to making healthy choices for myself and my family.

If you've been following the action items at the end of each chapter, you have been slowly adding new habits, better choices, and healthier options to your routine. If you haven't, I highly encourage you to go back through the book and start practicing those action items, making them your own. To help you get started, here is a general outline of what an average day looks like for me. Keep in mind that I am a busy mom, running several online businesses, maintaining a household and a homestead, and taking care of my family. I know the meaning of tired, I have experienced overwhelm, and I run a tight household budget. No excuses. I have been there, done that, and know where you're coming from. And, I'm here to say that it CAN be done. The hardest part is getting started, changing your mindset and approach, and gaining the knowledge. Throughout this book, you have that part down. Now, to move on to the next phase: Putting it all together!

An Example Day

An average day for me looks something like this:

I like to get up early before the rest of the household awakes. Granted, I am more of a morning person, and not everyone wakes up chipper and ready to attack the day. If you're not a morning person, don't let that be an excuse. First thing after getting up, I recite my affirmations for the day while I drink 16 oz of water, sometimes with lemon, sometimes with cayenne pepper, sometimes plain. I generally like to measure out my water for the day in a gallon glass jar, so I can easily visualize how much I need to drink and where I stand throughout the day in my water consumption. That way I always get enough water consumed to fully support my body.

AND GOD SAID:

Proverbs 16: 3

Commit to the Lord whatever you do, and your plans will succeed.

AND GOD SAID:

John 16: 23

In that day you will ask nothing of me. Truy, truly, I say to you, whatever you ask of the Father in my name, he will give it to you.

Then I take some time for prayer and meditation. I shoot for 30 - 45 minutes at least, but depending on the day, this is sometimes more like 15 minutes. Either way, I try to make this time a priority.

Before waking the rest of the household, I drink 8 oz of green juice (spinach, kale, wheatgrass, spirulina, chlorella, etc). I used to juice my own, but now I use Organifi Green Juice. It saves time, tastes great, and is economical for what it contains. I sometimes also add collagen, Organifi Red Juice, Aloe Vera Juice, Coconut Water, and/or some kombucha (homemade) for added nutrients and energy.

At this point, everyone else wakes up and I prepare for them a healthy breakfast. Breakfast generally consists of a garden fresh salad, soup or stew, an egg dish of some kind, lentils, or leftovers. Occasionally, I'll make my daughter's favorite: Einkorn Pancakes with Pure Maple Syrup. (See Recipes) I like to enjoy an herbal tea while we have our brief family time in the morning. When choosing recipes and meals, be aware that we are a product of our culture and it is through cultura dictates that breakfast must be unhealthy cereals or pastries. Breakfast can be anything, and in our home, we love choosing hearty breakfasts that give us the energy we need for the day.

After my husband leaves for work and my daughter is dropped off at school, I take 20-40 minutes for some fun exercise. This might be a brisk walk, some aerobics, weights, or what I like to call "cleansercise": where I do a blitz clean on the house, with some jammin' music, that gets my heart rate up and cleans the house at the same time! Anything that serves a dual purpose in a busy lifestyle is a bonus in my book!

Then I drink another big glass of water, so I can be sure to stay well hydrated.

Now it's time to get to work. The rest of the day, other than lunch, until my daughter gets home from school, is spent on working my businesses. For lunch, I like to have a good wholesome meal, since I find my digestion does better with a good wholesome breakfast and a light dinner. For lunch I may throw some fish or an organic chicken breast into the toaster oven, with some veggies on the side, or I'll do a quinoa salad, lentil salad, or other salad. I heard it said once for optimum

216

gestion, we should eat breakfast like a king, lunch like a queen, and dinner like a
auper. I find this philosophy to work very well for me.

hroughout the day, I always have my water bottle handy, taking sips often. I
so have healthy snacks handy like seeds, nuts, fruits, and veggies, and I enjoy a
ass of kombucha.

ter my daughter gets home from school, we take some time for homework and
ores, and sometimes have a healthy snack. This is when I head out to the
arden to tend what needs tending, pull a few weeds, and harvest the goodies.
ur animals get fed, and we collect the eggs from the chickens.

nner, I try to keep simple and light...because by now I'm usually ready to relax a
tle bit. Soups and stews are some of my favorites. Not only are they super
elicious and full of nutrients, but I can often throw the ingredients in the slow
oker or power pressure cooker in the morning so I don't have to worry about
king time to cook dinner in the evenings. In the online support group
ww.TheologenicDiet.com), I share a video about my favorite kitchen tools to
ake your life easier when transitioning to a healthier lifestyle, and the power
essure cooker is right up there near the top of the list!

ter dinner, we make sure to turn off any and all technology at least 2 hours
efore bedtime. We also have some herbal tea, Organifi Gold Juice, and/or
agnesium supplement about an hour or two before bed. My daughter and I like
read together before bed. Sometimes we read separate books, and sometimes
e read to each other from the same book. It is a time I cherish.

egardless of what your schedule looks like, what your budget may be, how much
ne you have, or your current health situation, you can incorporate the
eologenic Diet principles into your life. I believe that God never intended for
od to be such a challenge in our lives. The Garden of Eden was a paradise, with
the perfect foods we needed. Then, with a single bite of one forbidden fruit,
e world changed forever. But the foods from that paradise are still available to
. As with anything in our lives, God gives us choices. Through His abounding
ve, we have the freedom to make decisions for every aspect of our lives,
cluding what we eat. And, whether intentionally or unintentionally, every choice
e make has consequences on our health, either good or bad. Now that you are
med with the knowledge from this book, what will you decide? How will you
ed your children? What difference will you make to yourself and to those
ound you? I believe in you! And God is with you.

AND GOD SAID:

Revelation 21: 5

And he who was seated on the throne said, "Behold, I am making all
things new."

AND GOD SAID:

Romans 8: 26

In the same way, the Spirit helps us in our weakness. We do not know what we ought to pray for, but the Spirit himself intercedes for us through wordless groans.

What works for you

What works for me may not be the perfect solution that works for you, and that is what is so great about God's design. We are all different, yet throughout history, the Bible still applies to you and me and offers us invaluable tools, guidelines, and wisdom. What you see and experience when you read the Bible may be different than anyone else around you, but you are still growing in Christ each time you read the verses and turn the pages. What you see and experience from the scriptures about diet, health, and nutrition are no different. It is up to you to take the information offered here and prayerfully apply it to your life.

I used to think I was doing just fine. I was living the typical life, eating out a lot, working hard, under a great deal of stress, and focusing my priorities on my career. I thought I was happy, but I wasn't sleeping well, had horrible hormonal issues with very painful monthly cycles, dealt with the weight roller coaster constantly, no energy...especially in the afternoons, and often had uncomfortable skin issues. I thought all these things were "normal" and just part of being a woman, or getting older.

After making the key lifestyle changes outlined in this book, I continue to be amazed at the transformations in myself and my family. My monthly cycles are now nothing more than a minor inconvenience with no pain. I have abundant energy and a clearer mind. As a result, I get so much more done each day. I sleep deeply. My skin issues all cleared up. I no longer have seasonal allergies. I almost never get sick.

My daughter, who at the time of writing this book, is 11 years old and was pretty much raised on these principles. To this day she has never needed or taken prescription antibiotics and also almost never gets sick. And that's the best part of all, in my opinion. I am raising her to understand what it means to eat healthy and make better choices. She loves healthy foods, knows how to turn to things like essential oils and herbs when needed, and she loves the Lord. She even just wrote her own book, called *Healthy Habits for Kids* where she shares some of her experiences with other kids to teach them about making better choices at an early age. (www.HealthyHabitsforKids.com)

What you experience will be unique to you. I encourage you to seek professional counsel, if needed, especially if you are dealing with a major health concern. But most of all, just get started. Knowledge is the first step, but taking action is where you will reap the rewards. The concepts are simple:

1. *Focus on consuming foods that contain light energy.*
2. *Breathe deeply.*
3. *Drink more water.*
4. *Consume the right kinds of salt.*
5. *Soak your grains, and only use whole ancient grains that man has not destroyed or modified.*
6. *Enjoy lots of greens, fruits, and vegetables.*
7. *Only eat the right kinds of meat, prepared according to God's law.*
8. *Enjoy dairy that is certified A2 Beta Casein.*
9. *Limit sweets.*
10. *Focus on healthy fats.*
11. *Get enough probiotic foods to support the gut.*
12. *Periodically fast, cleanse, and detox.*
13. *Get enough sleep & rest, and take time for yourself.*
14. *Move your body regularly and get your heart-rate up.*
15. *Pray continually, live in faith, and turn your stresses over to God.*

Adopting these steps will change your life forever.

Notes:

Notes:

Chapter 18: Resources

It is my hope and prayer that you have found the information in this book insightful and beneficial. As you have absorbed the concepts, some may have been familiar to you and others may have been new. Any new idea takes some time to assimilate into your habits and routines.

To make things smoother for you as you transition to a Theologenic Lifestyle, we have created an online support program that guides you through all the concepts of this book with interactive videos, coaching, and a community of support. To find out more, enroll in our individual program at www.TheologenicDiet.com, or to enroll in our church study group program, visit: www.TheologenicLife.com.

Other resources available to you include our *Theologenic Diet Cookbook, Ditch Candida Cookbook,* and *Theologenic Diet for Kids.* Your kids will also love *Healthy Habits for Kids,* a fun and informative book written by my daughter Megan (at age 11) from a kids perspective on developing healthy habits. These and other books are available at www.HealthyHomesteadLiving.com.

For more in-depth coaching on preparing healthy meals, join our Living Foods Academy, where we teach you everything you need to know about making healthy foods according to God's plan for you. Whether you are brand new to the kitchen or a seasoned chef, you will find valuable insight into the world of fermented foods, nourishing broths, preparing grains, making sourdough, making your own dairy products, and so much more. Check it out at www.TheLivingFoodsAcademy.com.

I also include in this chapter some additional resources you may find beneficial. All resources, products, and recommendations are offered strictly for your benefit. I get no monetary gain by mentioning any of the products listed, and I personally use each and every one of them regularly. I encourage you to do your own research and find options that work best for you, your health, your budget, and your tastes.

Additional Reading:

Healthy Habits for Kids by Megan Olivia Austin. 2018. Maddix Publishing.
The Ultimate Guide to the Daniel Fast by Kristen Feola. 2010. Zondervan Publishing.
The Maker's Diet by Jordan Rubin. 2013. Destiny Image Publishing.
Healing Oils of the Bible by Dr. David Steward. 2015. Care Publications.
Nourishing Traditions by Sally Fallon. 2001. New Trends Publishing.
What the Bible Says About Healthy Living. by Dr. Rex Russell. 1996. Regal Books.

Self Heal by Design. Barbara O'Neill. 2015. Bang Printing.
Einkorn: Recipes for Nature's Original Wheat. Carla Bartolucci. 2015. Clarkson Potter.

Cultured Foods and Ferments:

Healthy Homestead Living: Educational website found at
   HealthyHomesteadLiving.com
Cultured Food Life, Donna Schwenk: Starter cultures, recipes, and how-to's found
   at CulturedFoodLife.com
Cultures for Health: Starter cultures, recipes, guides, and support found at
   CulturesForHealth.com

Essential Oils:

I love essentials oils, yet too often I see them being used incorrectly. Be sure to only use the best quality essential oils of pure, therapeutic grade, from a reputable company. Not all essential oils are created equally, and not all companies adhere to quality standards. The essential oil industry is self-regulated, therefore choose a reputable company who openly discloses sources and regulatory procedures.

Cleaning Without Chemicals

Norwex, found at Norwex.com, has a selection of quality microfiber cleaning
   products that effectively clean without the use of chemicals. I love these
   products and they make cleaning so much easier.
Soap Nuts are actually a dried berry that comes from the *Sapindus mukorossi* tree
   in the Himalayas. These berries contain high amounts of saponin, a
   natural cleaner that is particularly effective at gently and naturally
   cleaning laundry. The residue easily washes away, leaving no harmful
   chemicals on your clothing, and is much safer for septic systems. Soap
   nuts can be found from many different suppliers online.

Natural Healing and Holistic Care

Himalayan Salt Lamps: Himalayan Salt Lamps have been shown to reduce the
   possible risks associated with technology in the home. Personally, I find
   them a beautiful addition. We purchased our lamps from
   SpiritualQuest.com.
Infrared Saunas: Saunas are a wonderful way to relax and detox. If you have
   the space and the budget, you can now get your own personal infrared
   sauna. I love mine, and combine the power of the sauna with Himalayan
   Salt Bricks and Essential Oils for a truly cleansing and immune boosting
   experience.

Einkorn Grains:

Jovial Foods: Jovial Foods is one of the worlds premier sources for quality Einkorn flour and wheat. Their website, www.JovialFoods.com, also offers some great tutorials and recipes to help get you started.

Bulk Foods

Buying healthy foods in bulk, whenever possible, is one way to save. I like visiting local farmer's markets, buying meat directly from the farmers as a whole, half, or quarter, and participating in local co-op or CSA (Community Supported Agriculture). Here are a few websites that also carry bulk options:

Vitacost.com
ThriveMarket.com

Supplements

Even when eating healthy, sometimes we need a little additional supplementation to get all the required vitamins, minerals, and trace nutrients our body needs. Supplements are big business with very convincing marketing. In choosing supplements for you, I encourage you to consult your healthcare provider, then look carefully at the ingredients, sourcing, and sustainability of the products. A few that I use regularly include:

Organifi Green, Red, Gold Juice: For years I would make my own green juices every morning. I would grow the wheatgrass, juice it...along with other great ingredients, and then have to clean the juicer. Although this is wonderful nutritionally, I love the convenience, flavor, and nutrient density of Organifi. I rarely go a day without it any more. Best tasting green juice on the market! **www.OrganifiShop.com**. Use coupon code: HEALTHYHOMESTEADLIVING for a discount on your first order!

Shakeology: Made by Beach Body, these shakes are delicious and loaded with superfoods. Enjoying a shake or smoothie is the perfect option for those days when I don't have time, need an extra boost of energy, or want to make sure I'm getting a balanced meal. Find it at www.TeamBeachbody.com/Shakeology

Swedish Bitters: Consuming bitters at the end of meals containing meat help stimulate digestive enzymes. I use Swedish Bitters, and their website also has many other great herbs and resources.

Juice Plus+: It's not always easy to make sure we get enough fruits and vegetables each day, especially during the winter months when there are less options available in fresh form. To ensure my body gets those important nutrients and life energy, I take JuicePlus+. Learn more about their kids program, too, where your kids can get their yummy chewables for free at www.JuicePlus.com.

Chapter 19: Recipes

Whether you are a seasoned chef or just getting started in the kitchen, exploring new recipes is a fun way to get excited about following the Theologenic Diet and Lifestyle. Included in this chapter are a few simple and delicious recipes to help you get started. Visit my homestead website at www.HealthyHomesteadLiving.com for other cookbooks and resources to help you get started.

For additional ideas for recipes to try, most Mediterranean Diet Cookbooks and a few Paleo Cookbooks have some good options, just be aware that these programs have a few variances in their recommendations. When in doubt, always look at how much life energy is in the dish, and how much dead foods, toxic ingredients, or modified components may be included. Stick with life energy choices, and avoid those unhealthy options that will rob you of your health.

When grocery shopping, as a general rule of thumb, concentrate most of your time on the outside aisles and avoid the center. In most stores, the outside is where you will find the fresh produce, meats, dairy, and frozen items, with the center primarily consisting of your processed foods. This is just a general guideline, however, as there are still foods to avoid on the outside aisles, and a few good choices in the center.

Most importantly, have fun with this new adventure. Even if you don't like to cook at all, you can successfully adjust your lifestyle to a healthier, biblically-based one. I was at a conference one time with a man in our group who was in his 80's and who looked and acted like he was more like 45! I asked him his secret, and he told me that he makes health his hobby. What brilliant advice! Since then, I have made health my hobby, making a point to enjoy learning, trying new recipes, sampling new herbs, experimenting with new essential oils, and experiencing new holistic approaches to healing. When "Health is Your Hobby," all this becomes an adventure with amazing lifelong results.

The following pages are some great recipes to help get you started. My grandmother, Margaret, was an amazing cook who made everything from scratch. She grew up in a time when pre-packaged foods and modern conveniences weren't an option. Many of the recipes included here came from what I learned from her, or what I adapted from her old wooden recipe box that was passed down to me. I hope you enjoy them. Recipes, she always said, are meant to be individualized. So feel free to adjust them to your preferences and have fun in the kitchen as you embark on this new journey of health.

AND GOD SAID:

3 John 1: 2

Dear friend, I pray that you may enjoy good health and that all may go will with you, even as your sould is getting along well.

Breakfasts

Egg dishes like Fried Eggs, Poached Eggs,
    Omelettes, Quiche, Scrambled Eggs
Oatmeal (real rolled oats, not instant)
Einkorn Pancakes
Muffins made with Einkorn Flour
Quinoa-based recipes
Granola with sprouted grains
Soups and Stews
Lentil dishes
Quinoa dishes
Rice dishes
Smoothies and Green Juices
Leftovers

Lunches/Dinners

Vegetable-based dishes. Look for recipes
    that don't have meat as the main course
Salads
Fish and vegetables
Chicken or Turkey and vegetables
Taco Salad
Steak or Roast with vegetables
Einkorn Pita Bread filled with your favorite
    vegetables, tuna salad, chicken
    salad, lentil salads, or quinoa salads
Sourdough Einkorn sandwiches
Soups and Stews
Smoothies

Snacks

Fresh fruits and Vegetables
Soaked Nuts, Seeds, Nut Butters
Granola with sprouted grains
Sprouted grain crackers
Hummus
Guacamole with homemade tortillas
Fruit Leather
Cultured vegetables
Green Juices

Beverages

Water
Herbal teas
Kombucha
Kefir
Kvass
Homemade lemonade
Smoothies and Green Juices
Fresh vegetable juices
Fresh fruit juices (with the pulp)

*The possibilities are truly endless, and the variety of delicious choices just require a little adjustment in your personal paradigms. Experiment with new flavors, colors, and varieties of healthy vegetables, fruits, nuts, seeds, grains, and fats. You'll quickly find your favorites!

Almond Milk

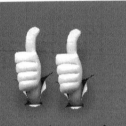

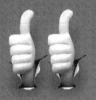

It's so easy making your own nut milks and the flavor is so much better than anything you can find at the store. In fact, the first time I made Almond Milk, we did a blind side-by-side taste test with my daughter and some of her friends...and the homemade won out hands down. Plus, you know there are no preservatives or filler ingredients. You do need some equipment for making nut milks including:
- Quality Blender such as Vitamix or Blendtec
- Cheesecloth or nut bag for straining

For a full tutorial on nuts, including making your own nut milks and nut butters with videos and printable instructions, check out our full Nuts course at HealthyHomesteadLiving.com.

1. Add to your Vitamix or other high powered blender the   following:
   - 1 cup nut of choice (almond, cashew, etc.)
   - 4 cups pure water
   - 1 tsp vanilla
   - ½ tsp stevia or xylitol (or to taste)
   - Pinch of Celtic Sea salt
2. Blend until smooth and milky.
3. Meanwhile, place a fine mesh strainer lined with cheesecloth or nut bag over a bowl.
4. Carefully pour nut milk into lined strainer and strain   completely to separate the pulp. Pulp may be dehydrated and ground into almond flour.
5. Transfer nut milk to glass jar and refrigerate or enjoy   immediately. Will store for about 1 week.

Note: Some settling or separation may occur while storing.
This is normal and your milk is still good. Just shake gently to re-mix. Never consume milk that smells "off". Nut milks are an excellent choice as a beverage or as a dairy substitute in many recipes as it is lower in calories and contains healthy fats.

Einkorn Pancakes

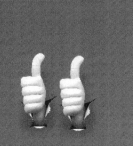

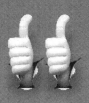

Einkorn flour comes from an ancient variety of wheat that hasn't been hybridized or altered. It is so delicious and is more easily digested than modern wheat. Einkorn does absorb liquids a little differently, though, so takes a little getting used to at first. Einkorn pancakes are a favorite in our house because they are so good, and incredibly filling. We like to make a few extras to have as leftovers for snacks.

1. Preheat flat skillet or pan to medium heat.

2. In a medium bowl, combine and beat:
   - 1 large egg
   - 1 cup milk (A2 dairy, almond, or other nut)
   - 3 Tablespoons melted butter
   - 1 teaspoon vanilla extract

3. In a separate bowl, combine and mix:
   - 1 ½ cups Einkorn All Purpose Flour
   - 1 Tablespoon baking powder
   - ¼ teaspoon sea salt

4. Combine wet and dry ingredients and whisk until well mixed.

5. Optional: Add mix-ins like blueberries, pecans, cinnamon, stevia-sweetened chocolate chips, etc.

6. Grease heated skillet with butter, ghee, or coconut oil.

7. Drop batter onto skillet using ¼ cup measuring cup.

8. Repeat to fill the skillet. Cook on first side until bubbles form in the middle and the edges are no longer sticky.

9. Flip to cook the other side, reducing the heat if necessary.

10. Repeat this process until all the batter is gone.

Serve with butter, ghee, maple syrup, homemade jam, or other favorite toppings.

Quinoa Breakfast Bowl

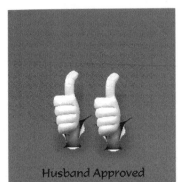

Husband Approved

Hubby says: "What a great combination of flavors and a change from the traditional oatmeal. I like this with extra coconut and a handful of fresh blueberries on top."

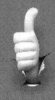

Kid Approved

Daughter says: "The texture of this took some getting used to, but the flavor is amazing."

Quinoa is an ancient grain that is super easy to make and lends well for a wide variety of recipes. This version is super hearty and filling and loaded with nutrients to get you going in the morning and keep you going!

Ingredients:

- 1 cup quinoa (sprouted)
- 2 cups water
- ¼ cup toasted unsweetened coconut flakes
- ¼ cup toasted slivered almonds, walnuts, or pecans
- 2 Tablespoons hemp seeds
- 1 teaspoon cinnamon
- 1 pinch cardamom
- 1 Tablespoon maple syrup or stevia to taste
- 1 dash sea salt
- Unsweetened (preferably homemade) almond milk (optional)

Cook 1 cup quinoa in 2 cups water for about 20 minutes or until quinoa has absorbed the water and is soft. Add remaining ingredients and mix together. Top with option al almond milk.

Inspired by The Whole Journey

228

Pumpkin Pie Baked Oatmeal

This recipe really makes the house smell amazing. The only trick is that you have to remember to soak your grains the night before. Pretty soon, recipes like this will be common for your new way of looking at food so it'll become part of your routine. If you are avoiding sugar, you can substitute the maple syrup for stevia.

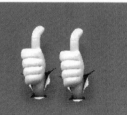

Husband Approved

Hubby says: "This is so delicious and very filling. It makes a great breakfast when I have to work because I don't get hungry until lunch."

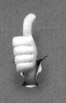

Kid Approved

Daughter says: "I like the flavor, but the texture isn't my favorite."

The night before:

In a large bowl, combine:
- 2 ½ cups rolled oats (organic and non-gmo)
- ¼ cup Einkorn berries or steel cut oats
- 2 tablespoons apple cider vinegar (with the mother)

Pour water over the mixture until covered. Stir and soak overnight.

In the morning:

Preheat oven to 350 and grease a 9x13 inch baking dish.
Drain the oat mixture in a fine mesh sieve and rinse with water.
In a large bowl, combine:
- 1 cup milk
- 1 ½ cup pumpkin puree
- 2 pastured eggs, lightly beaten
- 2 tablespoons melted butter
- ½ cup maple syrup
- 1 tsp baking powder (aluminum free)
- 2 tsp vanilla
- 2 tsp ground cinnamon
- ½ tsp ground ginger
- ¼ tsp ground nutmeg
- 1/8 tsp ground cloves

Mix thoroughly and combine with oat mixture.
Pour into baking dish.
In a small bowl, combine:
- 2 tablespoons coconut flour
- ¼ teaspoon ground cinnamon
- 1 tablespoon maple syrup

Sprinkle over the top of the oatmeal and bake for 30 minutes.
Serve warm.

Nourishing Bone Broth

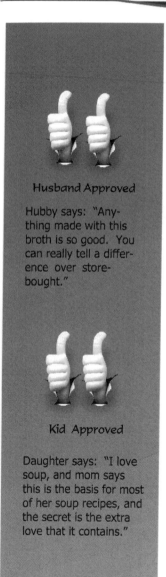

Husband Approved

Hubby says: "Anything made with this broth is so good. You can really tell a difference over store-bought."

Kid Approved

Daughter says: "I love soup, and mom says this is the basis for most of her soup recipes, and the secret is the extra love that it contains."

Bone broth is one of my favorite super-foods because it is loaded with so much good nutrition, is easy and economical to make, and creates the foundation for such a wide variety of delicious recipes. Excellent for immune support, bone and joint health, heart heath, skin health, brain health, and the list goes on. Make a big batch at once, and preserve what you don't use right away for efficient cooking. Use the guidelines offered here for chicken broth, turkey broth, fish broth, or beef broth. For more detailed information about how to make and preserve broth, including tutorial videos, check out our Nourishing Broths course in the Living Foods Academy at **www.HealthyHomesteadLiving.com**.

1. First, you will need **bones**. Best will be a variety of bones from a quality and organically raised animal, fish, or fowl. Broth is economical to make so it is recommended to get the best quality bones you can find. If possible, include feet, neck, and bones with tendons for the best broth.

2. Broth also contains a combination of **vegetables and herbs**. The classic combination, called a *mirepoix* in French cuisine, includes carrots, celery, and onions. You can add anything else that might be in your garden or maybe wilting in your refrigerator (broth is a great use for those veggies a little past their prime) such as:
  a. Root vegetables like beets, turnips, parsnips, jicama, and celeriac
  b. Vegetables such as leek, tomato, peppers
  c. Sea Vegetables such as kombu, wakame, kelp
  d. Herbs such as parsley, rosemary, thyme, sage, cilantro, bay leaf, mint, oregano
  e. Spices and aromatics such as peppercorns, garlic, horseradish, ginger, turmeric
  f. Other additions such as mushrooms, lemon and/or lime wedges

The combination of vegetables, herbs, aromatics, and spices will affect the flavor of your final broth. Feel free to experiment and find the ingredients that work best for you.

We don't recommend adding starchy vegetables such as potatoes or corn to your broth as they may adversely affect the final broth. Save those ingredients for your

ecipe after the broth has been made. Also, don't add salt to your broth. Salt can be added
ater in your final recipe when you can better control the final flavor.

. All good broth will require the addition of small amounts of **vinegar**. The vinegar helps
xtract minerals from the bones. Any good vinegar will do, and the vinegar doesn't need to
e raw or contain the "mother" since you will be heating the broth enough to negate the
enefits of raw. Apple cider vinegar is the most common choice, yet wine vinegar, white
inegar, kombucha vinegar, or other vinegar you may have on hand will work fine.

. You will want to use clean, filtered **water** for your broth. Try to avoid water that may be
ontaminated with any chemicals like fluoride or chlorine, often found in most city tap
ater.

he crockpot and the electric pressure cooker are our favorite methods of preparing broth.
he key to good broth is a long, slow simmer...the longer the better...at very low heat to
void scorching. With a crockpot, we can safely get a good slow simmer over a 12 hour
eriod (or more) without hassle or worry. The crockpot is a fairly common household
ppliance these days, so it negates the need to purchase extra equipment to make your
roth. Be sure to start with a clean crockpot, check carefully for cracks or blemishes, and
nd a safe place to situate your unit during the long cooking process.

*If using a whole chicken, frozen is acceptable. Cooked bones, leftover from previous
ecipes (like a good rotisserie chicken) may also be used. When using cooked bones, be
ure to add a chicken foot or other additional bones for added nutrient value. If using beef
ones, roast the bones at 350 degrees for at least 20 minutes before preparing your broth.

. Place bones, vegetables, herbs, spices, and vinegar in the crockpot. (Frozen whole
nicken is acceptable with the crockpot method. If making broth with large vertebrate
ones such as beef, roast the bones for 30 minutes at 350°, turning once.)
. Fill with filtered water to cover the bones. Careful not to over-fill the crockpot.
. Place the lid on the crockpot.
. Plug in and set crockpot to the lowest possible setting or longest cooking time
epending on your unit.
. Cook for 6-24 hours.
. Unplug crockpot and cautiously remove lid, facing lid away from you to direct steam
way from your body.
. Carefully strain off broth, remove meat (if applicable). Broth and meat will be HOT!
. Allow broth to cool to room temperature or use in your favorite recipe.
. If not using right away, store strained broth as desired. You can preserve broth by
eezing, canning, dehydrating, or freeze-drying.

Best Chicken Vegetable Soup

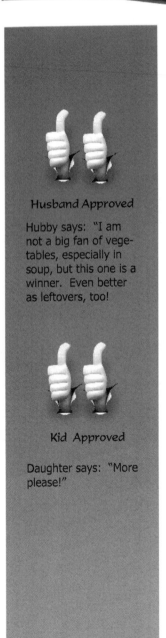

Husband Approved

Hubby says: "I am not a big fan of vegetables, especially in soup, but this one is a winner. Even better as leftovers, too!

Kid Approved

Daughter says: "More please!"

This is a favorite recipe in our household! Best when the vegetables are fresh from the garden, but frozen or canned will also do well. Add what ingredients you have and feel free to improvise. I lovingly call this recipe my "everything but the kitchen sink recipe." Even my husband, who doesn't love many vegetables and says he's not fond of soups, will gobble this one up.

Delicious when served with fresh baked sourdough bread!

1. Combine the following ingredients in a large stockpot and simmer on low for about 20 minutes:
   - 4 cups turkey or chicken bone broth
   - 1 medium zucchini, cut into ½ inch slices
   - 1 medium carrot, cut into slices
   - 1 rib celery, cut into thin slices
   - 1 chopped leek or sweet onion
   - 1 cup green beans
   - ½ cup lima beans
   - 3 Tblsp pearl barley
   - 3 Tblsp fresh or 1 Tblsp dried parsley
   - 1 tsp minced garlic
   - ¾ tsp pepper
   - ½ tsp dried oregano

2. Add the following ingredients and simmer an additional 10 minutes.
   - 2 cups cooked, diced turkey or chicken
   - 1 cup broccoli
   - ½ cup fresh or frozen peas (not canned!!!)
   - 1 cup whole kernel corn
   - Salt to taste

Ladle into your favorite soup bowls and enjoy!

Hungarian Mushroom Soup

I first had this recipe at a Soup Cook-off Contest at the local farmer's market. My vote went to the Shiitake Mushroom Farm who made this incredibly delicious soup. Easy to make, incredibly nutritious, reheats very well for amazing leftovers the next day, and is economical too. I recommend using smoked Hungarian paprika rather than regular paprika for extra flavor.

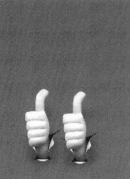

Husband Approved

Hubby says: "I didn't think I would like this recipe the first time I tried it, especially since I'm not usually a big soup fan, but this one is really good and very filling."

Kid Approved

Daughter says: "I love this soup. It's one of my   favorites."

1. Melt butter in a large pot over medium heat. Saute 4 cups
chopped onions until translucent.
2. Add 4 lbs fresh sliced mushrooms (especially good with shiitake) and saute about another 5 minutes or so.
3. Stir in:
    - 4 tsp dried dill
    - 2 T paprika
    - 2 T coconut aminos
    - 4 cups (1 quart) chicken or beef broth (homemade best)
4. Reduce heat to low, cover, and simmer for about 15 minutes.
5. Whisk together and add:
    - 2 cups whole organic milk
    - 3 Tablespoons Einkorn all purpose flour
6. Stir well to blend, cover and simmer another 10 minutes on low
heat, stirring occasionally.
7. Stir in:
    - 2 tsp Celtic Sea Salt
    - Pepper to taste
    - 2 tsp lemon zest (or zest from 1 large organic lemon)
    - ¼ chopped fresh parsley
    - 1 cup sour cream.
8. Remove from heat. Mix thoroughly until all ingredients are well
blended. DO NOT BOIL.

Inspired by Ozark Shiitake Farms

Cream of Whatever Soup

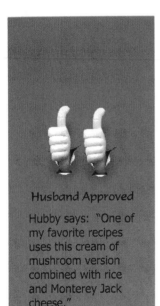

Husband Approved

Hubby says: "One of my favorite recipes uses this cream of mushroom version combined with rice and Monterey Jack cheese."

Kid Approved

Daughter says: "By itself I give it one thumb, but combined in different yummy recipes, this one gets two thumbs up."

Commercial canned cream soups are loaded with sodium and preservatives. This recipe came from an old Mennonite cookbook and works great as an easy way to make your own. Make up a big batch and preserve it for future use. Use in recipes calling for cream of mushroom, cream of chicken, cream of celery, cream of broccoli, etc.

Heat 3 Tablespoons of coconut oil in a saucepan on medium heat. Stir in 3 Tablespoons Einkorn flour (or you can use gluten free flour/almond flour/etc.) and keep stirring until the flour is golden and bubbly. Slowly whisk in 1 cup broth (homemade chicken, beef, etc.).

Turn down the heat and stir until the sauce is at the desired consistency. It should be thick and creamy.

Cream of Mushroom: Chop up ½ cup of mushrooms and saute in the oil before adding the flour. Continue in the recipe.

Cream of Celery: Chop up ¼ cup celery and saute in the oil before adding the flour. Continue in the recipe.

Cream of Chicken: Use chicken broth and add ½ cup chopped cooked chicken.

Creamy Cheese Soup: After adding the broth, add 1 cup shredded cheddar cheese. Stir until well blended. This works great for homemade Mac and Cheese. Just add your favorite sprouted grain cooked elbow macaroni.

Butternut Squash Soup

This is such a flavorful recipe and one I love to fix in the fall when the days are just starting to get crisp. Butternut squash can be prepped ahead of time by peeling and dicing, then freezing for quick, grab-and-go convenience. Look for turkey bacon that doesn't contain any nitrates or nitrites and if possible, make your own chicken broth. Grandma Margaret always said that the quality of the recipe is only as good as the quality of the ingredients. So true!

Ingredients:
- 1 large butternut squash, peeled and cut into chunks
- 3 whole carrots, peeled and cut into large chunks
- 1 ½ tablespoons coconut oil, melted
- ½ lb turkey bacon, chopped
- 1 small onion, chopped
- 1 small apple, chopped
- 2 cups chicken broth
- 1 cup full fat coconut milk
- 1 tsp Celtic or Himalayan Pink salt
- 1 tablespoon cinnamon
- 1 tablespoon nutmeg
- ½ cup raw pumpkin seeds, toasted

Instructions:
1. Preheat oven to 350 degrees F.
2. Toss squash and carrots with coconut oil and arrange on a baking dish. Roast uncovered for 35 minutes or until tender.
3. In a large stock pot or Dutch oven over medium heat, cook turkey bacon until crisp. Remove bacon and set aside for garnish.
4. Add onion and apple to the pot and saute until tender, about 5 minutes. If the onions and apples stick to the pan, add a little butter, ghee, or coconut oil.
5. Add the roasted squash and carrots to the pot and stir. Add broth and coconut milk and bring to a boil, stirring often.
6. Remove from heat.
7. Use an immersion blender, carefully blend the soup until smooth.
8. Season with salt, cinnamon, and nutmeg.
9. Serve warm, topped with turkey bacon and toasted pumpkin seeds.

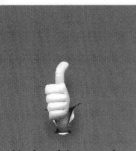

Husband Approved

Hubby says: "The bacon and pumpkin seeds really add to the flavor and texture of this soup. Very filling."

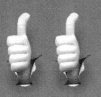

Kid Approved

Daughter says: "This soup is like eating at a fancy restaurant, but at home!"

Onion Soup Mix

This is a staple item in my pantry since it's so good and make recipes just sing. If you garden, make your own dried onion flakes in your dehydrator...or buy the ingredients in bulk and save. Great for dips, sauces, and dressings but also incredible on steaks or in soups. Have fun with this one, especially since it's LOADED with healthy.

Ingredients:

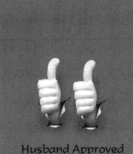

Husband Approved

Hubby says: "Hard to judge just the dry mix, but I know I love everything made with it so it must be two thumbs up."

- 1 cup dried or dehydrated onion flakes
- 2 tsp onion powder
- 2 tsp garlic powder
- 1 tsp celery powder
- 1 tsp black pepper
- 2 tsp Celtic Sea Salt
- 1 tsp turmeric

Mix all ingredients and store in an airtight glass jar. I usually make
this in big batches at once so I always have plenty on hand. About ¼ cup of the above mix is equivalent to 1 packet of the commercial onion soup mix.

** Add ¼ cup to 2 cups beef broth for a quick and easy French Onion Soup
**Add ¼ cup to yogurt or sour cream for a super veggie dip
**Excellent on roasts, steaks, lamb, or other meats as a rub.

Kid Approved

Daughter says: "I especially love this one as a dip or on steak."

Inspired by Wellness Mama

Beef Pot Roast

I grew up on a farm with lots of beef cattle so just say "Pot Roast" and I start salivating. Tender and juicy, pot roast is almost like comfort food to me. The best part, is left-overs make some fantastic soups...like try adding it to our Hungarian Mushroom Soup for a delicious beef version (recipe on previous page). You may not have many left-overs, though, as good as this recipe is! You can make it in the oven in a roasting pan, but I recommend using the Crock Pot or Power Pressure Cooker for extra convenience and time savings.

1. In a roasting pan, Slow Cooker, or Pressure Cooker, combine:
   - 1 beef roast (any cut, but we especially like Chuck Roast)
   - Celtic Sea Salt and Pepper rubbed into beef roast
   - 4 cups (1 quart) beef broth or water (the broth will be extra rich,
   add nutrients, and make a great au jus or gravy
   - 1 large onion, chopped
   - 2 cloves of garlic, minced
   - 1 T balsamic vinegar (trust me!)
   - 1 sprig fresh rosemary (optional)

2. If you are roasting in the oven preheat to 325º, then when oven is hot, place roasting pan on center rack, covered, and roast for 2
hours and 15 minutes. If using a Slow Cooker, cook on low for
6-8 hours. If using a Power Pressure Cooker, cook on high pressure for 35 minutes then allow pressure to equalize on its
own (about another 10 minutes)
   - Add additional root vegetables like carrots, turnips, parsnips,
   beets, and rutabaga.
   - Add fresh mushrooms
   - Add 1 quart of diced tomatoes
   - Replace fresh rosemary with fresh thyme
   - Double the garlic

Note: To make a gravy, remove and strain 2-3 cups of the broth after cooking. While still very hot, add ½ Cup Einkorn flour per 4 cups of liquid used and stir briskly until thick. Serve immediately.

Inspired by a recipe from Grandma Margaret

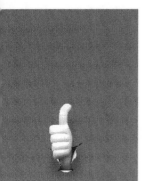

Husband Approved

Hubby says: "Delicious and filling. I like this one with lots of gravy on top and some melted pepper-jack cheese."

Kid Approved

Daughter says: "I remember having this for dinner even before I started doing to school. It's so good, especially with a baked sweet potato."

Pecan Dusted Cod

This recipe is a great choice if you're wanting something yummy that feels a little "fancier" yet without the fuss or mess. Super fast to make and crazy easy...plus it tastes so good. The combination of cod with pecans makes a delightful dish any time of day.

Ingredients:

- 4 cod fillets, 6 ounces each
- 2 T Greek yogurt
- 4 T chives, chopped
- 1 tsp horseradish
- 1 zest from lemon
- ½ cup pecans, very finely chopped

Directions:

1. Preheat oven to 425 degrees.
2. Place cod in a lightly-greased, shallow baking dish.
3. In a small bowl, mix the Greek yogurt, chives, horseradish, and
lemon zest. Season mixture with sea salt and pepper.
4. Cover cod evenly with mixture and top with pecans.
5. Bake for 18-20 minutes or until the fish is done, and the crust is
golden and crunchy.

Inspired by The Whole Journey

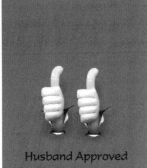

Husband Approved

Hubby says: "This is a delicious choice if you're in the mood for seafood."

Kid Approved

Daughter says: "I loved the flavor, but the texture of the fish with the crunchy nuts wasn't my favorite. Tasted good."

Grilled Chicken Marinade

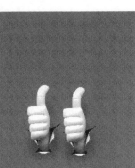

My mom used to make this recipe when I was a kid and it was always a hit. I'm not sure where she got it, as is often the case with handed down recipes. You can use a grill pan on the stove or a panini press, but the best flavor comes from an outdoor grill. Make a few extras so you have leftovers as this chicken is amazing on salads or used in other recipes.

Husband Approved

Hubby says: "You would never guess when eating this chicken that it was prepared with vinegar. The flavors are amazing."

Ingredients:

½ cup water
½ cup Apple Cider Vinegar
2 Tablespoons Avocado or Extra Virgin Olive Oil
1 teaspoon Basil
1 Tablespoon Coconut Aminos
½ teaspoon Garlic Powder
1 teaspoon Celtic Sea Salt
2 teaspoons Pepper
¼ teaspoon Celery Salt

Combine ingredients in a bowl with a tight sealing lid. Add 6-8 Chicken Breasts and stir to coat. Marinate for at least 6 hours or overnight.

Preheat grill or grill pan until hot. Remove chicken from the marinade and cook thoroughly on both sides until meat is no longer pink.

Kid Approved

Daughter says: "This chicken is really good, especially dipped in mom's homemade ranch dressing."

Watermelon Feta Salad

Watermelon is one of my favorite fruits, and this recipe is so incredibly refreshing and delicious. You really have to try this one when the watermelons are in season and the days are long and hot. If you don't want to heat up the house with the oven, use the grill or a toaster oven.

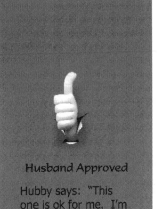

Husband Approved

Hubby says: "This one is ok for me. I'm not a fan of balsamic but it's very refreshing and full of flavor."

Kid Approved

Daughter says: "I can't get enough of this salad! It has so many of my favorites...watermelon, feta, sprouts, and balsamic!"

1. Preheat oven to 350 degrees and adjust the rack to the middle position.
2. In a bowl, gently combine:
   - 1 cup crumbled feta cheese
   - 1/8 teaspoon red chili flakes
   - Juice from ½ an orange
3. Pour into an oven proof dish and drizzle with olive oil.
4. Bake for 20 minutes until just golden brown on the tops.
5. Meanwhile, in a medium bowl, toss to combine:
   - 1 ¼ cups fresh sprouts (greens, mung beans, celery leaves, etc.)
   - ¼ cup fresh mint leaves
   - Juice from 1 lemon
6. Slice watermelon to about ½ inch thick large slices.

To serve:

Place watermelon slices on salad plates. Divide warm feta on top of each piece of watermelon. Evenly divide the salad mix and place on top of the feta. Drizzle with:
   - Balsamic Vinegar.

Inspired by Deliciously Organic

Savory Quinoa Bowl

I came up with this recipe one day when I was low on groceries and needed a quick dinner. Made from staple pantry items, it is super quick and easy to make. Good warm or cold, as a main dish or a side, and feeds a crowd easily and economically. I love taking this one to potlucks or family gatherings and it makes a great conversation starter, because everyone will ask you for the recipe once they try it.

Ingredients:

2 cups water
1 cup quinoa (I use tricolor mix, but you can use white, red, black
     or a combination)
¾ cup homemade salsa (or use a good sugar-free salsa you like)
2 sweet onions
Handful of fresh spinach or kale
1 box Chicken Sausage (we use Applegate Farms. Look for a good
     brand without nitrates or sugars added)

Directions:
1. Bring water to boil. While water is heating, rinse quinoa in cold water. Best to use sprouted if possible.
2. Once water is boiling, add quinoa and reduce heat to simmer. Cook 10 minutes or so until almost done.
3. Meanwhile, cook sausage. Chop into small pieces once cooked.
4. Chop onion. In a separate pan, heat butter, ghee, or coconut oil on medium heat and saute onion until tender. Lower heat and caramelize until quinoa is done.
5. Once quinoa is soft and fully cooked, add salsa, onion, sausage and stir to combine flavors.
6. Add spinach or kale and heat a few more minutes until wilted.
7. Salt and pepper to taste.

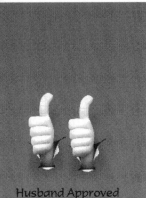

Husband Approved

Hubby says: "I didn't think I liked quinoa until I tried this recipe. Very good."

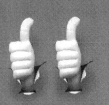

Kid Approved

Daughter says: "I love this recipe, even though mom tries to sneak spinach in it."

Homemade Mac n Cheese

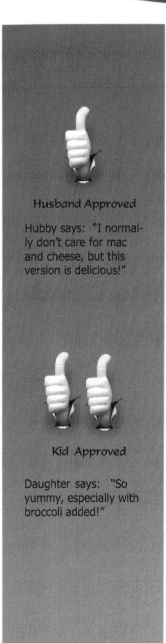

Husband Approved

Hubby says: "I normally don't care for mac and cheese, but this version is delicious!"

Kid Approved

Daughter says: "So yummy, especially with broccoli added!"

Who doesn't love a good Mac and Cheese, but the commercial boxed or canned versions are just not ideal for a healthy choice. This recipe is always a hit with the kids and you can rest assured that they are getting a wholesome meal that nourishes. Serve as a side dish to fish, chicken, or roast and some steamed vegetables. The sauce can be made ahead of time if needed. The sauce is also excellent on diced, cooked potatoes.

In a medium pan, saute until soft:
- 1 small onion, finely chopped
- ¼ cup (1 stick) of butter

Blend in:
- ¼ cup Einkorn All Purpose flour
- 1 tsp Celtic or Himalayan Pink Sea salt
- ½ tsp dry mustard powder

Mix well, then gradually add:
- 1 ½ cups A2 milk

Reduce heat to medium/low and cook, stirring constantly until thickens. Add:
- 2 cups shredded cheddar cheese

Meanwhile in medium pot, bring 6-8 cups water to boil. Add:
- One box sprouted quinoa elbow macaroni

Reduce heat and simmer about 7 minutes or until noodles are el dente. Drain noodles, and return to pot.

Pour thickened cheese sauce over noodles and stir to combine. Serve warm.

Variations:
- Add steamed broccoli and/or steamed mashed cauliflower at the end and stir to combine.
- Top with chopped diced tomatoes or homemade salsa.
- Add diced grilled chicken breast, tuna, or ground beef.
- Top with shredded fresh parmesan and bake at 350 for 15 minutes.

Homemade Pita Bread

Making your own bread products with Einkorn flour is fun, satisfying, and so delicious! This Pita bread is super versatile and can be used for a wide variety of meals. Be careful not to let the pitas get too brown when baking or they may lose some of their softness.

Ingredients:
1 cup warm water (around 100 degrees F)
½ tsp dry active yeast
4 cups All-Purpose Einkorn Flour
1 ½ tsp fine sea salt

Instructions:
1. In a small bowl, combine the water and yeast until the yeast is dissolved. In a separate bowl, combine flour and salt.
2. Add the yeast mixture to the flour mixture and mix together. Knead the dough with your hands until it holds together.
3. Transfer to a clean work surface and knead for 1 minute or until the dough is smooth and a bit sticky. Place the dough back in the bowl, cover tightly, and let proof for 1 hour.
4. Lightly flour a clean work surface. Divide the dough into 10 equal pieces. Cover the pieces with plastic wrap until you are ready to shape them.
5. Roll each piece of dough into a 6 inch round. Dust parchment paper with Einkorn flour and place round dough on it. Cover with another piece of parchment paper. Repeat the process until all pieces are shaped. Let rest for 45 minutes.
6. Preheat oven to 400 degrees. Place a baking sheet in the oven to preheat the baking sheet.
7. Remove the heated baking sheet from the oven and place 2-3 pitas on the sheet. Bake for 4-5 minutes until they have puffed up but not browned. Wrap baked pitas in a clean kitchen towel while you continue to bake the rest.
8. Serve warm or store in a sealed container for up to 3 days. May also be frozen for up to 1 month.

Inspired by Carla Bartolucci

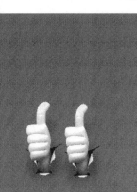

Husband Approved

Hubby says: "Fresh from the oven is best. I especially love these filled with marinara and cheese for a pizza pita."

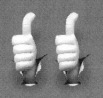

Kid Approved

Daughter says: "These are so good. My favorite is warm pitas with a little bit of butter and mom's homemade jam."

Einkorn Tortillas

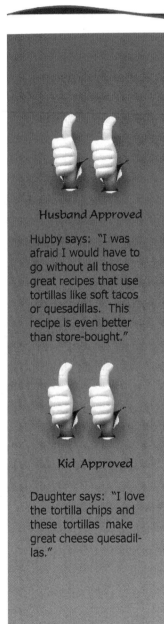

When we were first transitioning to ancient grains, one of the staples our family loved and ate regularly were tortilla Homemade tortillas are super easy to make, and once you experience the difference in flavor between homemade an what you used to eat, you'll never look back. Super versa tile, and can also be made into tortilla chips by just cutting into wedges, brushing with olive oil and seasonings of choice, and baking at 350 for 22 minutes.

Ingredients:
- 4 cups all-purpose Einkorn flour
- 1 ½ tsp Celtic or Himalayan Pink Sea Salt
- ½ tsp baking powder (Aluminum Free)
- 1 cup warm water, at about 100 degrees F
- 3 tablespoons extra virgin olive oil

Instructions:

1. In a large bowl, combine dry ingredients. In another bowl, combine water and oil. Add the wet mixture to the dry mixture and mix as much as you can.
2. Knead the dough in the bowl until it forms a ball. Cover and let rest for 15 minutes.
3. Lightly flour a work surface and transfer the dough to it. Knead the dough for 1 minute until smooth.
4. Heat a cast iron skillet or griddle on medium hea for 10 minutes.
5. Divide the dough into 12 equal pieces and form into balls. Lightly dust the ball with flour. Using rolling pin, carefully roll out each piece to an 8 inch diameter round, adding more flour as needed.
6. Place the tortilla on the hot griddle. The dough should lightly sizzle, but not burn. Cook for abou 45 seconds on each side until done.
7. Serve warm or store in airtight container for up t 2 days. Tortillas also freeze well.

Inspired by Carla Bartolucci, Jovial Foods.

Jalapeno Popper Dip

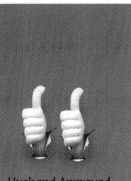

This recipe is a family favorite and a common request for holidays and get-together's. Serve with sweet potato chips, fresh vegetables slices, or homemade crackers. I sometimes make this just for the leftovers as my husband's favorite Sweet Potato Quiche is when I add this Jalapeno Popper Dip to the egg mixture before baking...or add it to scrambled eggs for a special treat. It's also wonderful added to your lettuce wraps. Best served warm, but can also be served cold. If you don't like "heat", be sure to remove all the seeds and membranes from the jalapeños. Look for quality turkey bacon without nitrites or nitrates.

Note: I tend to gravitate towards European cheeses as they will have a higher likelihood of having A2 beta casein than American varieties, if you can't find certified A2 in your area.

Ingredients:
- 6-8 slices of turkey bacon, cooked crispy and diced (or add extra if you love extra bacon flavor)
- 2 (8 oz.) Packages of cream cheese, softened
- 1 cup homemade mayonnaise or crème fraiche
- 4-6 jalapeño peppers, de-seeded and chopped fine
- 1 cup cheddar cheese, shredded
- ½ cup mozzarella cheese, shredded
- ¼ cup diced green onion
- ½ cup shredded fresh parmesan cheese

1. Preheat oven to 350º.
2. Combine all ingredients except parmesan cheese in a medium bowl.
3. Stir well to fully combine.
4. Transfer to an oven safe shallow dish. I use a glass lasagne pan.
5. Top with shredded parmesan cheese.
6. Bake for 20-25 minutes or until cheese is bubbly and well melted.
7. Allow to cool slightly and serve warm.

Inspired by Christina Cooper

Italian Mushrooms

Mushrooms make a great quick snack. Saute them plain with a little butter then salt to taste, or try adding some additional flavors like what we offer in this recipe. Don't use canned mushrooms as the texture is just not as good as fresh. Any mushroom variety will do, but we especially like shiitake if they are available.

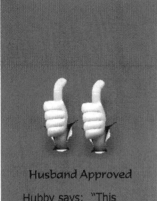

Husband Approved

Hubby says: "This recipe makes a great snack, but is also really good as a topping on eggs."

Ingredients:

- 1 lb mushrooms, sliced
- 2 tablespoons coconut oil, butter, or ghee
- 1 tablespoon fresh basil, chopped
- ½ teaspoon garlic powder or 1 clove minced garlic
- Sea Salt and Pepper to taste

Instructions:

1. Heat oil or butter in a skillet over medium heat.
2. Add mushrooms and saute until mushrooms are slightly browned.
3. Top with seasonings and stir to coat.

Serving ideas:

Serve alone as a snack.
Serve as a side dish.
Serve over eggs or as a filler for omelettes.
Mix with softened cream cheese and sour cream for a mushroom dip.
Serve as a topping for steak.

Kid Approved

Daughter says: "I love mushrooms and this recipe is really good, especially when mom serves them with sauerkraut and fresh tomatoes."

Homemade Gummy Snacks

Kids, young and old alike, seem to love gummy fruit snacks but so often they are loaded with sugar, toxins, and preservatives. Our version is super easy to make, a fun project with the kids, and has only wholesome, healthy ingredients. The gel sets up quickly, so you'll want to prep well ahead of time before beginning the recipe. Have all your tools and ingredients ready.

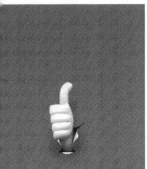

Husband Approved

Hubby says: "I'm not usually a fan of gummy snacks, but these are very flavorful and sweet."

Kid Approved

Daughter says: "I could eat these until my tummy hurts."

1. Puree in a blender or food processor **1 cup fruit** of choice until completely smooth. Fresh or frozen are fine, and you can even use applesauce if you want. A favorite in our house is fresh strawberries.
2. Measure out **1 cup kombucha or fruit juice** and have ready.
3. Boil **½ cup water**.
4. Place **½ cup cool wate**r in a small bowl or jar. Add **½ cup gelatin powder** and stir quickly to create a paste.
5. Quickly add the ½ cup boiling water to the paste and stir briskly. This should form a thick but stirable liquid.
6. Add **¼ cup honey**, 1 cup kombucha or fruit juice, and pureed fruit. Stir well with a whisk or use an immersion blender.
7. Very quickly pour the mixture into molds or a creased glass baking dish or other greased dish and allow to cool in the fridge for 2-3 hours.
8. Carefully remove from molds or cut into bite-sized chunks.
9. Store in the fridge in an airtight container for 1-2 weeks (if you can get them to last that long.)

Inspired by Wellness Mama

Chia Seed Pudding

Chia seeds are so good for the digestion. When soaked, they become gelatinous that offers bulk, fiber, and prebiotics for the gut. This recipe is loaded with Omega 3, antioxidants, and calcium, making it a great breakfast, snack, or dessert. Start with the basic recipe, then make it your own by adding fresh fruit, nuts, or spices.

In a blender or food processor, combine:
- 2 cups nut milk (coconut, almond, cashew, etc)
- ½ cup Chia Seeds
- ½ teaspoon Vanilla Extract
- ¼ cup (or less) sweetener of choice such as honey or maple syrup (or use stevia)
- ¼ teaspoon cinnamon

Blend until smooth (one to two minutes). Pour the mixture into a jar or glass container and place in the refrigerator for at least 4 hours or overnight to let the mixture gel and thicken.

Add fruit or flavoring to taste. Fruits and flavors can be added during the blending stage if desired.

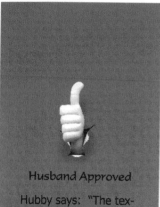

Husband Approved

Hubby says: "The texture of this took some getting used to, but I love the flavor, especially with lots of fresh blueberries and pecans."

Kid Approved

Daughter says: "Delicious. My favorite is strawberry and banana."

Zucchini Brownies

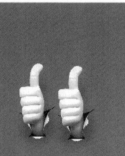

Brownies are our go-to choice for birthdays since they are cake-like and delicious. This recipe is so incredibly moist and fudgy...you'd never guess it was actually good for you! Cacao powder is different than cocoa powder in that it is less refined and loaded with beneficial magnesium! Top with Homemade Ice Cream (recipe on the next page) for a truly decadent treat.

1. Preheat oven to 350º and line an 8x8 baking pan with parchment
paper. Set aside.
2. In a large bowl or Stand Mixer, whisk together:
   - 1 cup finely shredded zucchini (it should look like puree)
   - 6 T melted butter
   - 2 T melted coconut oil
   - 1 large egg
   - ½ cup honey or Cup-for-Cup Stevia (or equivalent stevia)
   - 1 T vanilla
3. Add slowly, folding through slowly until just combined:
   - ¾ cup almond flour
   - 1/3 cup cacao powder
   - 1 tsp baking powder
   - ¼ tsp Celtic Sea Salt
4. Fold in ¼ cup Stevia-Sweetened Chocolate Chips
5. Pour into prepared pan.
6. Bake for 30 minutes or until the brownies spring back when gently touched.
7. Allow to cool; cut into squares.

Inspired by Cafe Delites

Homemade Ice Cream

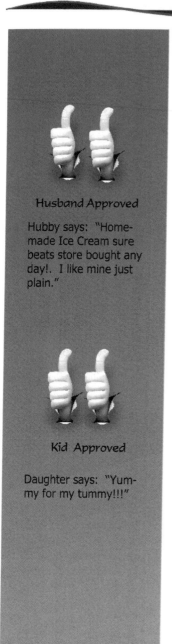

Ice Cream is such a special treat any time of year for young and old alike. The key is to use A2 Beta Casein Milk and Cream. You do need an Ice Cream Maker of some kind, and we recommend the Cuisinart version because you don't need any salt or other accessories. Since Ice Cream is a frozen dish, limit how much or how often you have it if you are having digestive issues, since cold foods add extra stress to the digestive system. Look for high quality cream from grass-fed organic antibiotic-free A2A2 Beta-Casein cows. Grandma Margaret always said the quality of a recipe is only as good as the quality of the ingredients and this especially holds true with Ice Cream!

1. Pre-freeze the ice cream bowl if using a Cuisinart Ice Cream
Maker.
2. Remove ice cream bowl from freezer, assemble machine, and
add:
- 2 cups Heavy Cream
- 1 cup Whole Milk
- 1 T vanilla
- ½ tsp liquid stevia (vanilla flavored is especially good)
3. Turn on machine. Ice cream will be ready in about 15-20 minutes.

Variations:
- Add ½ tsp cacao powder, mixed with 1 tsp melted coconut oil for chocolate ice cream.
- Add 4-5 drops of Food Grade Peppermint Essential Oil for peppermint ice cream.
- Add 3-4 drops of Food Grade Lemon Essential Oil and grated Lemon Zest for lemon ice cream.

Sleepy Time Tea

I modified this recipe from a version by Maria Treben in her book *Health Through God's Pharmacy*. This combination of herbs really does the trick for encouraging a deep sleep and reducing stress or anxiety. For some people, these herbs are pretty potent, so I wouldn't recommend planning any activity or operating any equipment after drinking it. Generally considered safe for ages 2 and up.

1. In a large glass bowl, combine the following herbs:
   - 50 grams Cowslip
   - 25 grams Lavender
   - 10 grams St. John's Wort
   - 15 grams Hops Flowers
   - 5 grams Valarian Roots
   - 15 grams Holy Basil
   - 15 grams Chamomile Flowers
2. Gently mix and store in an airtight container out of direct sunlight.

To brew the tea, steep 1 tsp herb mixture per cup of very hot water (not boiling). Cover and infuse for 3-5 minutes. Add honey or stevia if needed for taste. Drink 1-2 hours before bedtime.

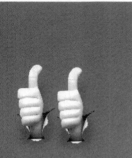

Husband Approved

Hubby says: "This tea tastes really good, especially with a little bit of honey, and really works! I was surprised the first time I tried it how hard I slept."

Kid Approved

Daughter says: "This tea smells so good and tastes good too! I like mine just lightly warm...not too hot, in my favorite mug."

Homemade Laundry Soap

I spent years experimenting to find a laundry soap that I loved yet had peace of mind while using it. My husband comes home from work filthy, sweaty, and stinky...so I need something STRONG and EFFECTIVE yet non-toxic and gently. Norwex has a great brand of laundry soap that we like, and Soap Nuts do a pretty good job. Here is the best homemade version I found to work the best, and it's easy to make and economical too!

2 parts washing soda (not baking soda, and available at most
     grocery stores)
2 parts Borax
1 part bar soap, grated fine or powdered in a food processor
    (I like Fells Naptha, Dr. Bronner's Pure Castile Bar Soap,
    or a homemade lye soap)
(Optional) Essential Oils of choice

Combine ingredients and store in an airtight jar or closed container. Use 2 Tablespoons per load of laundry.

Safe to use in HE Machines.

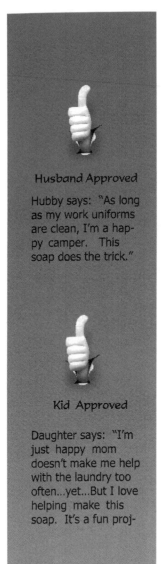

Husband Approved

Hubby says: "As long as my work uniforms are clean, I'm a happy camper. This soap does the trick."

Kid Approved

Daughter says: "I'm just happy mom doesn't make me help with the laundry too often...yet...But I love helping make this soap. It's a fun proj-

References

Chapter 1:

1: www.photoniclighttherapy.com

Chapter 2:

2: Moran, Tim. "The Amazing Healing Power of Oxygen". September 25, 2014. http://www.sandiegouniontribune.com/news/health/sdut-amazing-healing-power- oxygen-2014sep25-story.html

3: Burroughs, John. The Breath of Life. 2017. Pinnacle Press http://www.oxygen-review.com/human-body.html

4: Inogen. "Low Oxygen Symptoms: Signs You May Not Be Getting Enough Oxygen". October 7, 2013. https://www.inogen.com/blog/signs-your-loved-one-may-not-be- getting-enough-oxygen/

5: Clark, Steve. "The 'Breath' of God and Gifts of the Spirit." July 2014. http://www.swordofthespirit.net/bulwark/june2014p2.htm

6: Lobo, Patil, Phatak, and Chandra. "Free radicals, antioxidants and functional foods: I mpact on Human Health." 2010. https://www.ncbi.nlm.nih.gov/pmc/articles/PMC3249911/

7: Friesen, Kristi. Boost Your Immune System with Antioxidants. July 2015. https://www.openhand.org/blog/boost-your-immune-system-antioxidants?gclid=EAIaIQobChMI4oHK3PPI2AIVkTuBCh3b5QSYEAAYASAAEgJjwPD3wE

7: Clark, Stephen. Charismatic Spirtuality: The Work of the Holy Spirit in Scripture and Practice. 2004 Servant Books. http://www.swordofthespirit.net/bulwark/june2014p2.htm

Chapter 3:

8: Brown, Valerie Cheers. "Who Many Times is "water" Mentioned in the Bible and how Significant is It?". March 2015. https://cultureandplacesboutiquetravel.wordpress.com/2015/03/25/how-any-times-is-water-mentioned-in-the-bible-and-how-significant-is-it-by-valerie-own-cheers/

9: "How is Water Delivered?" http://www.freedrinkingwater.com/water-ducation3/32- water-tab-water.htm

10: Postman, Andrew. January 2016. "The Truth About Tap." https://www.nrdc.org/stories/truth-about-p?gclid=EAIaIQobChMIvpev26jd2AIVD6ppCh3EuAb_EAAYASAAEgJNZPD_BwE

11: The Restored Church of God. "How Clean Are You?" Volume 9, Issue 6. https://rcg.org/pillar/0906pp-hcay.html

12: Russell, Rex M.D. What the Bible Says About Healthy Living.

Chapter 4:

*13:   Renee, Janet. "What is the Importance of Water & Salt".
    http://healthyeating.sfgate.com/importance-water-salt-body-homeostasis-
10409.html
*14: Ford, Mike. "Salt". November 2002.

https://www.cgg.org//index.cfm/fuseaction/Library.sr/CT/ARTB/k/758/Salt.htm
*15:   Kresser, Chris.   "Shaking up the Salt Myth". April 2012.
    https://chriskresser.com/shaking-up-the-salt-myth-history-of-salt/
*16 Lackey, Kimberly.   "15 Side Effects of Table Salt."
    https://www.curejoy.com/content/15-harmful-health-effects-of-table-salt-
to-worry-about/
*17: Gundersen, Melissa.   "5 Different Types of Salt and How They Affect
Health".   https://bembu.com/different-types-of-salt/
*18: Leonard, Jayne. "10 Compelling Reasons to have a Himalayan Pink Salt Bath
Today."   January 2016. http://www.naturallivingideas.com/himalayan-
pink-salt-bath/
*19: Axe. "Pink Himalayan Salt Benefits that Make it Superior to Table Salt."
    https://draxe.com/pink-himalayan-salt/

Chapter 5:

*20: Gilkerson, Luke. "5 Ways Modern Wheat is Different than Biblical Wheat."
November   2013. https://www.intoxicatedonlife.com/2013/11/07/5-ways-
modern-wheat-different-biblical-wheat/
*21:   Dnews. "Why You Should Probably Stop Eating Wheat." 2012.
    https://www.seeker.com/why-you-should-probably-stop-eating-wheat-
1766312242.html
*22: "Grains." 2018.   Cooking with the Bible.
    http://cookingwiththebible.com/reader/Default.aspx/GR3410-4106/lore/
*23: "Grains of truth about Wheat Production and Consumption." 2004. Wheat
Foods Council. http://www.californiawheat.org/uploads/resources/282/wheat-
prod.-&-consumption.pdf
*24:   Reinhart, Peter. "Sprouted Whole Grains."
https://wholegrainscouncil.org/whole-g rains-101/whats-whole-grain-refined-
grain/sprouted-whole-grains
*25: Bartolucci, Carla. Einkorn Recipe Book.
*26: Hagin, Kenneth.   "Christ: The Bread of Life."
http://www.rhema.org/index.php?option=com_content&view=article&id=1014:ch
rist-the-bread-of-life&Itemid=140
*27:   Forerunner.   2007.
    https://www.cgg.org/index.cfm/fuseaction/Library.sr/CT/RA/k/1358/Ask-
It-Will-Be-Given.htm
*28: "The Lord's Table: The Meaning of Bread."
    https://fullcontactchristianity.org/2010/02/21/the-lords-table-the-
meaning-of-bread/

9: Davis, William M.D. "Wheat Belly." 2014. Rodale Books, New York, NY.

apter 6:

0: Szalay, Jesse. 2015. "What are Phytonutrients?"
        https://www.livescience.com/52541-phytonutrients.html
1: Axe, Josh. "Chlorophyll Benefits." https://draxe.com/chlorophyll-benefits/
2: George Mateljan Foundation. "Sea Vegetables." 2017.
        http://www.whfoods.com/genpage.php?tname=foodspice&dbid=135
3: Roizman, Tracey, D.C. "What Benefits Can you Get from Eating Mushrooms?"
    17.
        http://healthyeating.sfgate.com/benefits-can-eating-mushrooms-4412.html
4: Sabaratnam, Wong, Naidu, & David. "Neuronal Health- Can Culinary and
    edicinal
        Mushrooms Help?" 2013.
        https://www.ncbi.nlm.nih.gov/pmc/articles/PMC3924982/
5: USDA Department of Agriculture. "Organic Standards." 2018.
        https://www.ams.usda.gov/grades-standards/organic-standards
6: "What does it Mean to be a Fruitful Christian?". 2015.
        https://www.gotquestions.org/fruitful-Christian.html

apter 7:

7: Russell, Rex. M.D. "What the Bible Says About Healthy Living." 1996. Regal
    oks,
        Ventura, California. (page 76-77)
8: Colbert, Don, M.D. "What Would Jesus Eat." 2002. (pages 49-50).
9: United Church of God. "What Does the Bible Teach About Clean and Unclean
    eats?"
        2008.
0: Maguire, Jessie. "Grass-fed vs. Regular Beef – What's the Diff?". 2017.
        https://well.org/healthy-body/grass-fed-beef-and-regular-beef/
1: Arnarson, Atli. PhD. "Why Processed Meat is Bad for You." 2017.
        https://www.healthline.com/nutrition/why-processed-meat-is-bad.
2: Cole, Karlsson, & Sage. "Are Processed Meats More Unhealthy Than Other
    d
        Meats." www.center4research.org/processed-meats-dangerous-red-meats/
3: Fallon Morell, Sally. "Nourishing Broth." 2014. Grand Central Life & Style,
        Hatchette Book Group. New York, NY.
4: Schwartz, Richard, Dr. "When Eating Meat was a Sacrifice."
        https://www.myjewishlearning.com/article/when-eating-meat-was-a-
    crifice/

apter 8:

5: Fallon, Sally. "Nourishing Traditions, Revised Second Edition." 2001. New
    ends

Publishing, Inc. Washington, D.C. page 33.
*46: https://www.betacasein.net/
*47: Rubin, Jordan. "The Maker's Diet." 2013. Destiny Image Publishers, Inc. Shippensburg, PA. pages 160-161.
*48: Beck, Leslie. "Is it Healthier to Drink Grass-fed or Organic Milk?" https://www.theglobeandmail.com/life/health-and-fitness/health/is-it-healthier-to-   drink-grass-fed-or-organic-milk/article20726402/
*49: Palmer, Linda Folden. "Baby Matters". 2001. Lucky Press, LLC. Lancaster, OH.
*50: Schwenk, Donna. "Cultured Food for Life." 2013. Hay House, Inc. New York, NY.

Chapter 9:

*51: Golden Blossom Honey. "Honeybee Facts." http://www.goldenblossomhoney.com/education_bees.php
*52: Sangor-Katz, Margot. "You'd Be Surprised at how many Foods Contain Added Sugar."   New York Times. 2016. https://www.nytimes.com/2016/05/22/upshot/it-isnt-easy-to-figure-out-which-foods-contain-sugar.html
*53:   https://bamboocorefitness.com/not-so-sweet-the-average-american-consumes-150-170-pounds-of-sugar-each-year/
*54: Schaefer, Anna and Yasin, Kareem. "Experts Agree: Sugar Might Be as Addictive as   Cocaine". October 2016. https://www.healthline.com/health/food-nutrition/experts-is-sugar-addictive-drug#1

Chapter 10:

*55: "Olive Oil." http://www.land-of-the-bible.com/content/olive-oil
*56: Gunners, Kris. 2017. "Saturated Fats, Good or Bad?" https://www.healthline.com/nutrition/saturated-fat-good-or-bad#section2
*57: "7 Reasons to Eat More Saturated Fat". 2009. https://articles.mercola.com/sites/articles/archive/2009/09/22/7-reasons-to-eat-more-saturated-fat.aspx
*58: "20 Benefits of Coconut Oil" 2015. https://draxe.com/coconut-oil-benefits/
*59: "Why Butter is a Superfood." 2012. https://empoweredsustenance.com/5-reasons-why-butter-is-a-superfood/

Chapter 11:

*60: Sass, Cynthia. MPH, RD. "The Real Benefits of Apple Cider Vinegar." 2016. http://www.health.com/nutrition/apple-cider-vinegar-benefits
*61: Newcomer, Laura. 2012. "13 Reasons Tea is Good for You." http://healthland.time.com/2012/09/04/13-reasons-to-love-tea/
*62: Collins, Martin. Forerunner Commentary. "Symbolism of Wine." https://www.bibletools.org/index.cfm/fuseaction/Topical.show/RTD/cgg/ID/3831/Wine-Symbolism-of-.htm

Chapter 12:

63: AromaTools. Modern Essentials: A Contemporary Guide to the Therapeutic Use of Essential Oils. 2015. Sixth Edition. Page 6-7.
64   Dr. Eric Z.   "The Truth about Gold, Frankincense, and Myrrh."
https://drericz.com/truth-about-gold-frankincense-and-myrrh/
65: AromaTools. Modern Essentials: A Contemporary Guide to the Therapeutic Use of Essential Oils. 2015. Sixth Edition. Page 96.
66: No data. We're skipping this number as a reference.
67:   Dr. David Steward, Ph.D.   Healing Oils of the Bible.   2015.   Care Publications, Marble   Hill, MO. Page 32.
68:   Dr. David Steward, Ph.D.   Healing Oils of the Bible.   2015.   Care Publications, Marble   Hill, MO. Page xvii.
69:   Dr. David Steward, Ph.D.   Healing Oils of the Bible.   2015.   Care Publications, Marble   Hill, MO. Pages 28-30.
70:   Dr. David Steward, Ph.D.   Healing Oils of the Bible.   2015.   Care Publications, Marble   Hill, MO. Page 151.
71: AromaTools. Modern Essentials: A Contemporary Guide to the Therapeutic Use of Essential Oils. 2015. Sixth Edition. Page 140.
72:   Dr. David Steward, Ph.D.   Healing Oils of the Bible.   2015.   Care Publications, Marble   Hill, MO. Page 33-34.
73:   Frawley, Donna.   "Herbs of the Bible."   Frawley's Fine Herbary.
http://jhawkins54.typepad.com/files/herbs_of_the_bible-frawley.pdf
74:   Karimi, Ali, Majlesi, Maedeh, and Rafieian-Kopaei, Mahmoud.   "Herbal Versus S   ynthetic Drugs."   Journal of Nephropharmacology.   2015.
https://www.ncbi.nlm.nih.gov/pmc/articles/PMC5297475/
75:   "What does it mean to be anointed?"
https://www.gotquestions.org/anointed.html

Chapter 13:

76: "Indoor Air Can Be Deadlier Than Outdoor Air, Research Shows."
https://www.cnbc.com/2016/04/22/indoor-air-can-be-deadlier-than-outdoor-air-research-shows.html
77: Chemicals of Concern. Norwex, Inc. 2017. www.norwex.bix

Chapter 14:

78:   https://www.mnn.com/health/healthy-spaces/blogs/student-science-experiment-finds-plants-wont-grow-near-wi-fi-router

Chapter 15:

79: "This is What Happens to Your Body When You Exercise". September 2013.
https://fitness.mercola.com/sites/fitness/archive/2013/09/20/exercise-health-benefits.aspx

Thank you for reading this book. It is my hope and prayer that you found it informative, beneficial, and life-changing in a positive way. If you enjoyed this book, we encourage you to tell your friends, share it on social media, talk about it in your church groups, and give it as a gift to those you love. The message I wrote within these pages is one of hope, health, and love, and through you we can better share this message with the world.

God Bless,

Rebecca Austin

Made in the USA
San Bernardino, CA
08 August 2018